TAKE IT OFF
AND KEEP IT OFF

A Behavioral Program
For Weight Loss
And Healthy Living

D. BALFOUR JEFFREY

ROGER C. KATZ

A SPECTRUM BOOK

PRENTICE-HALL, INC., Englewood Cliffs, N.J. 07632

Library of Congress Cataloging in Publication Data

Jeffrey, D Balfour.
  Take if off and keep it off.

  (A Spectrum Book) (Self management psychology)
  Bibliography: p.
  Includes index.
  1. Reducing.   2. Reducing—Psychological aspects.
I. Katz, Roger C., joint author.   II. Title.
RM222.2J43   613.2´5   77-4121
ISBN 0-13-882860-1
ISBN 0-13-882852-0 pbk.

© 1977 by Prentice-Hall, Inc., Englewood Cliffs, New Jersey 07632

A Spectrum Book

10 9 8 7 6 5 4 3 2 1

Printed in the United States of America

PRENTICE-HALL INTERNATIONAL, INC., *London*
PRENTICE-HALL OF AUSTRALIA PTY. Limited, *Sydney*
PRENTICE-HALL OF CANADA, LTD., *Toronto*
PRENTICE-HALL OF INDIA PRIVATE Limited, *New Delhi*
PRENTICE-HALL OF JAPAN, INC., *Tokyo*
PRENTICE-HALL OF SOUTHEAST ASIA PTE. Ltd., *Singapore*
WHITEHALL BOOKS LIMITED, *Wellington, New Zealand*

Contents

v

C

D

E

F

G

H

Preface

In a step-by-step way this book describes a self-help program for losing weight permanently. The major premise is simple: Being overweight is the result of too much eating and too little exercise. Since eating and exercise are habits people *learn* to do, they are things that people can learn to do *differently*. Our emphasis, therefore, is on ways to bring about habit change—slowly, surely, and, most important, in a way that you can live with for good.

If you're reading this book in search of an effortless cure or another crash diet that will finally work, you'll probably be disappointed. You'll find no such cure. However, you will learn how your behavior operates and what you can do to change it. By breaking the habits that have put excess weight on and kept it there, you can make the overweight problem a thing of the past.

Beginning in Chapter 3, we call upon you to become an *active participant;* in this chapter we ask you to assess your present commitment and readiness. Our recommendations for losing weight are accompanied by specific tasks for you to do, goals for you to work toward, and feedback methods to continuously see how well your goals are achieved. Many of the tasks require you to take a close look at such behavior as your food buying, your snacking, and your physical activity habits. Other tasks spell out what you can begin to do to change those habits permanently: using food exchange diets, enlisting the positive support of friends and family, learning to reward desired changes as they occur. Above all, you have to be committed to do things differently. Weight loss will never occur without the *doing.*

In making our recommendations, we have intentionally avoided either setting rigid time frames or prescribing rules that you *must* follow. Because new learning occurs at different rates in different people, *try out* the recommendations and procede through the tasks at a pace you feel comfortable with. Ideas alone won't change a thing. But new ideas can become a catalyst for new behaviors and make a lasting difference.

Our weight loss program is not just another passing fad; it is based on substantial evidence derived from carefully conducted research and experience. We've been heavily influenced by the findings of a number of prominent medical and behavioral scientists, people like Dr. Albert Stunkard, Dr. Jean Mayer, Dr. Richard Stuart, and Dr. Mike Mahoney—all of whom have contributed greatly to the understanding and treatment of overweight problems. On the other hand, we've added many procedures based on our own research and clinical experience with overweight clients. In the final analysis, we've tried to bring together recent clinical and research findings into a single, readable book—one conducive not only to self-directed learning but to safe and effective weight loss also.

Although the book is mainly intended for people who have

struggled with the "expanding waistline syndrome" and who want to do something about it, it can also be used by students, professional therapists, and researchers alike. Students in such fields as psychology, sociology, nursing, social work, nutrition, physical education, and medicine—anyone interested in practical applications of behavioral principles to such a health problem as obesity—will find the material appropriate. For the therapist or counselor, the book is designed to serve as a useful patient education tool to be supplemented with appropriate personal counseling. For example, the program can be used in outpatient clinics, in weight loss groups, or for parents of overweight children (Chapter 13). Health and behavioral researchers may also be interested in the book for purposes of comparative analysis and evaluation—activities we welcome and encourage.

We would like to thank the many people who helped immensely in bringing the book to completion. First and foremost, special thanks go out to Dr. Carl Thoresen whose incisive feedback and constructive suggestions were invaluable. Similarly, Ms. Lynn Lumsen, editor for Spectrum Books at Prentice-Hall, also deserves special thanks for her encouragement and support in making the book possible, as does Mrs. Rashel Jeffrey for her continuous patience and understanding while the book was being prepared. Thanks are extended to illustrator, Holle Brian, for her drawings. We also want to thank our friends and families for their suggestions and support. Finally, we would like to thank our students and clients whose names are too numerous to mention individually but whose contribution was immense and greatly appreciated.

1

Some Facts About Being Fat

In the United States and other Western countries, approximately one out of every three persons is obese. Yet, ironically, most of us know little about what causes or cures obesity. Obsessed with a healthy, lean appearance and repulsed by ugly fat, we often rely on folklore and myth in search of that "good thin life." As a result, we spend millions of dollars annually on get-slim-quick plans, magical gimmicks, gadgets, potions, shots, and pills—some complete with glowing testimonials and money-back guarantees.

Unfortunately, none of them work very well. The best of them promise too much and help some people lose weight for only a while. The worst are downright dangers to your health—physically and mentally.

If you want to take off weight and keep it off too (or help others do the same), you should know what you're up against.

No matter what you may think, or would like to believe, permanent weight loss means, above all, *permanently changing your eating and activity habits.* Changing habits takes a lot of time, effort, and patience. But the task can be made easier by a better understanding of the "loyal opposition" in a kingdom of quick foods, fast eating, and big portions. To make the task as easy as we can, we'll begin with what today are considered *facts* about being fat.[1]

THE DIFFERENCE BETWEEN BEING OVERWEIGHT AND OBESE

"Overweight" and "obese" are a couple of terms that you'll be seeing throughout this book, and they need defining. Although both may describe the shape you're in, they don't necessarily mean the same thing.

Being *overweight* means you weigh more than most people of the same sex, age, height, and body build as you. To find out if you're overweight, make a comparison of your own weight against statistical norms, which are usually contained in a weight chart. Norms show the normal, or average, weight of a large sample of similar people. If you weigh more than the figure shown for your sex, age, height, and build, you may consider yourself overweight. Remember, however, these norms tell you only how your weight compares with the average weight of others like you.

The term *obese* refers to the fat content (adipose tissue or cells) of your body. All of us have some fat on our bodies and need it to provide a source of energy and to protect our vital organs. But people are obese when they have an excess of body fat, which can be determined in a number of ways—as you'll

---

[1]We admit there's still much to be studied about the problems of obesity. These facts may change as we learn more.

soon see. Obesity therefore depends on how much fat we carry and not how much we weigh.

The distinction between being overweight and being obese is important, because you can be one without being the other. For example, an Olympic class shotputter or weightlifter is almost certainly overweight. Compared to the "average" person, his age and height, he probably weighs considerably more. But he is not necessarily obese. The added weight is probably due not so much to surplus fat as to a lot of well developed muscles. Similarly, though a person with a very sedentary life style may not be overweight (that is, an individual's weight may fall in the normal range for a particular reference group), *he or she could still be obese.* That's right—even though your weight is essentially normal, too much of it may be surplus body fat.

Though the difference between being overweight and obese is important, a person whose weight greatly exceeds a statistically derived "normal," "desirable," or "ideal" range is probably obese, as well as overweight. In many cases the two terms can be used interchangably.

HOW TO TELL IF YOU'RE TOO FAT

Although there are several ways to measure "fatness," some are better than others because they tell you more about the shape you're in. Let's explore a few of these measures, along with their advantages and disadvantages.

HEIGHT–WEIGHT CHARTS

One of the most common methods to find out if you're overweight is by means of a height–weight chart, like the one your doctor has used or the one in Chapter 4. Most of these charts are organized according to height and frame size (small, medium, large), and they show what your ideal weight should be depending on your size and stature. (Since you're comparing your weight to others' like you, the comparison is of course not really "ideal" in any sense of the word. As used here, the term actually means average or typical.) Weight charts are therefore used diagnostically: If your weight is more than twenty to twenty-five percent higher than your ideal weight, as shown on the chart, your doctor will very likely diagnose you as obese.

Although height–weight charts are a quick and easy test of your weight, they can also be misleading for rather complicated reasons, which boil down to the following four points:

First, the charts most commonly used today are derived from thousands of Metropolitan Life Insurance Company customers—people who do not necessarily represent a cross-section of America's population with its diversity of racial, ethnic, and socioeconomic groups. This information helps insurance companies know which type of person is most likely to get sick and die quickly and, thus, which types should be charged higher premiums. (In case you didn't know, overweight people are charged more!) For some of you, checking your weight against the ideal on the chart is like comparing apples and oranges. For a valid comparison you should be like the group upon whom the norms were based. And you may not be.

A second reason for being skeptical is that the information in weight charts may be outdated. What was normal twenty-five years ago may not be normal today. In the past few decades, dietary habits have changed rapidly. Standards of living have improved, making more food—including the "convenience" and "junk" variety—available to more people. New technology has eliminated the physical work from many jobs and recreational pursuits. Even cultural values about the attractiveness of being large or small vacillate as quickly as hemlines rise and fall. For example, the ideal weight of American males today is about fifteen percent higher than it was thirty years ago. Weight charts, like other normative, or average, information, need to be updated as norms change. Frequently they aren't.

Third, height–weight charts provide no precise rules to help you judge your frame size; whether your frame is small, medium, or large is left entirely to guesswork. What's your frame size? Is your torso long? Are your legs short? It is therefore possible for your ideal weight to vary by ten pounds or more depending on the frame size category you select.

Fourth, and perhaps most important, weight charts take only body weight into consideration. They indicate nothing about the real culprit, *individual differences in body fat.* As pointed out before, if you're overweight, you're not necessarily overfat; and conversely, if you're overfat, you need not be overweight.

ALTERNATIVES TO HEIGHT-WEIGHT CHARTS

To avoid the problems with height-weight charts and to obtain a more direct measure of fatness, several other methods to determine your proper weight have been developed. Many of them are easy to use, and they can provide a better measure of the shape you're in than weight charts alone.

The first is called a *mirror* (or *eyeball*) *test.* The way it works is simple. Take a good look at yourself, naked, in front of a mirror. What you see is what you are. The picture tells the story. In this case, if a lot of bulges, ripples, and soft flabby tissue are staring you in the face, it means you are too fat.

If the mirror test leaves you in doubt, there are other methods that rely on skinfold thickness. One of them is the *pinch test,* which determines the amount of surface skin fat that can be lifted free from the underlying soft tissue and bone. A good place to apply the test is to your tricep area. With your elbow bent and using your thumb and forefinger, gently pinch the *back* of your tricep midway between the elbow and shoulder. If you can lift away more than half an inch to an inch of flab, you probably have too much body fat. This conclusion is especially true if you're less than fifty years old.

Another related method is called the *ruler test,* which measures the amount of slope on your stomach while you are lying on your back. Here's how the test is done: Lie flat on your back, then place a twelve-inch ruler along the midline of your stomach so that it forms a line between the lower rib cage and the pelvic area. If the ruler lies flat so that it touches the lower rib and pelvic areas simultaneously, you're in good shape; at least you're not overloaded with fat around the midriff. If it can't touch the two end-points at the same time, the test indicates a surplus of body fat. (No fair sucking in your stomach!)

Several other tests for estimating body fat—such as X-ray or densimetric analyses where the body is totally submerged in water—are also available. But such tests require special equipment and a skilled professional. Certainly if, after such tests, a doctor advises you to lose weight for your own good health, it is in your best interest to follow such advice. If you want to learn more about these tests, see your doctor.[2]

All the tests and doctor's advice can tell you is whether your present weight is desirable or whether you've been victimized by creeping obesity. As helpful as the tests are, however, *you alone must decide on what kind of shape you'd like to be in.* Simply ask yourself, "Will I look better, and feel better if I lose weight?" The choice to lose weight is yours to make, and the commitment yours to build and develop.

---

[2]Other information is available in recent books on obesity, such as Mayer (1968) or Stuart and Davis (1972). The complete references can be found in the back of this book.

YOU ARE NOT ALONE

No matter who you are, if you're overweight and obese you've a lot of company. Fatness is a problem of epidemic proportions, a major public health problem in the truest sense of the word. Because nationwide estimates on the prevalence of overweight problems are relatively new, long-term, longitudinal comparisons are difficult. Nevertheless the proportion of overweight people appears to be higher now than it used to be. Easy modern living, mass media food advertising, the so-called agricultural revolution, and increasingly sedentary habits seem to be making the epidemic worse.

Though estimates of the number of overweight adults in this country vary according to the criteria used to make the diagnosis, the numbers range from forty to eighty million Americans. No matter how you look at it, that's a lot of people.

Figures compiled by the United States Public Health Service[3] are even more revealing: About thirty-five percent of all American men and forty percent of all American women forty years of age and older are at least twenty percent heavier than they should be. That's often considered obese. Such figures are not peculiar to Americans only; similar statistics have been obtained in England and other Western European countries.

Finally, let's not forget the children. As you'll see in Chapter 13, as many as one third of the youngsters in the United States are too heavy for their size and age. These obese children are very likely to remain obese, eventually becoming the next generation's overweight adults—unless something is done to stop it.

But as the problem has increased, so has the public's

[3]*Obesity and Health,* an undated monograph published by the U.S. Government Printing Office, Washington, D.C.

awareness of it. For example, a 1964 survey of Americans indicated that:

> . . . some 9.5 million said they were on diets, another 16.5 million reported they were watching their weight so they wouldn't gain, and still another 26.1 million expressed some concern about their waistlines. It is reasonable to conclude, therefore, that the ranks of the calorie-conscious add up to fifty-two million eaters. [Wyden, 1965, p. 1]

THE HIGH COST OF BEING FAT

Many people lose weight for cosmetic reasons. By losing weight they look better and feel better about their appearance. In this respect the payoff for dieting is relatively quick. But when you stop and think about the costs of being fat, there are many other *long-range* reasons for slimming down. Excessive weight is not only unattractive in our society; it is unhealthy, psychologically painful, and expensive.

HEALTH HAZARDS

Any doctor who encourages you to lose weight knows that being overweight increases the risk of serious diseases and ailments. What are some of these health hazards?

1. Cardiovascular Problems. Being overweight puts an extra burden on the heart, which has to work harder to pump blood through surplus fatty tissue. Obviously, the risk of heart attack increases under these conditions. Furthermore, if you're overweight you probably have a large supply of blood fat and cholesterol in your system. This condition can lead to arteriosclerosis (a blocking of the blood vessels by fatty deposits), together with high blood pressure (hypertension). These effects of obesity are often precursors to stroke and kidney disease.

2. Muscular and Skeletal Problems. Being overweight makes it hard to move around. It also puts an unnecessary strain on muscles and joints, which can lead to other complications such as arthritis (particularly in the knees) and lower back pain. When movement becomes painful, you learn to be less active. The resultant insufficient exercise weakens all your muscles, including the heart muscle. Thus a vicious cycle starts and keeps going.

3. Metabolic Problems. Diabetes, which is a failure of the body to produce the needed amounts of insulin to process sugar properly, is often preceded by obesity. In many cases this disease can be controlled by weight loss and better dietary habits.

Among pregnant women obesity is a particular problem. When the mother-to-be is markedly overweight during her pregnancy, there is a greater risk of toxemia (blood poisoning), complications during delivery, and stillbirth.

4. Earlier Mortality. Actuarial tables have been developed to estimate the normal life expectancy for people living in this country. Specifically, they show that obesity is associated with an increased mortality rate, particularly from heart-related illnesses. The plain fact is that staying fat increases your chances of dying sooner. Obesity can be literally as serious as life or death.

EMOTIONAL AND SOCIAL COSTS

Precise statistics on the prevalence of psychological problems in overweight people do not exist. Any information that is available should be interpreted cautiously because it does not necessarily represent the overweight population in general; that is, most fat people who end up in the statistician's folder by going to psychiatrists are the same ones who are emotionally disturbed. Whether the type of problems found in this *self-selected* group are also found in the total population of fat people is hard to know.

Nevertheless, like many popular myths, the idea that underneath the fat exterior lies a jolly "Santa Claus" personality is pure nonsense. The truth is that extra pounds can cause needless psychological pain, neurotic symptoms, and deep depression. As a matter of fact, there is reason to believe that obese people, compared to the non-obese, have more than their share of emotional difficulties. The differences are not always great, but they do exist.

For example, Albert Stunkard, a noted psychiatrist who has worked extensively with overweight people, reports that many of his patients suffer from "binge eating." They feel compelled to eat, and, when they do, they eat in a frantic, uncontrolled fashion.

Another frequent disturbance has to do with distortions in body image. Many overweight people perceive their own bodies as grotesque and ugly. They also attribute such perceptions to others, believing that onlookers view their bodies with utter disgust. When these feelings occur regularly, they're naturally upsetting and very often lead to still other hang-ups. Among them are anxiety and depression, which may come from the perceived threat of being unliked, embarrassed, or rejected as a friend. Whether the threat is real or imagined is probably irrelevant: A harmless remark, a caustic putdown, a casual glance, or a hostile stare are all apt to be interpreted personally. When they are, they perpetuate and confirm the negative feelings.

Other psychological problems found in overweight people have to do with self-esteem and self-confidence, both of which tend to be low. Better self-feelings can come about when unwanted weight is removed.

In addition to the psychological burdens of being overweight, adverse social consequences are involved. Fat people meet with difficulties in participating in active sports. They are often reluctant to join in social events.

Further, their employment opportunities are limited. Some jobs are just not suited for the overweight, such as in police and fire departments. In others the person may be the victim of hiring discrimination because of his or her weight; for example, recent cases involving such discrimination have occurred in the airlines industry. Some employers seem to have a built-in prejudice against fat persons, who, they may feel, lack self-discipline, or whose presence will detract from the youthful, energetic image the employer is trying to create. For whatever reasons, being overweight makes job finding more difficult and can also affect your chances for advancement or promotion after finding employment.

ECONOMIC COSTS

Finding and keeping a job is just one source of economic hardship. Others come from increased doctor bills, since the chances of sickness or accident seem to be greater among the overweight. For the same reason, life insurance premiums are also higher.

Overweight people pay tremendous sums every year on slimming aids and devices. Before 1972, when the federal government began regulating the sale and manufacuture of diet pills—the so-called appetite suppressants—there were at least seventy prescription-restricted drugs on the market. Many of them contained amphetamine, a substance with a real potential for physical and psychological dependence and abuse. One large drug company alone (Smith, Kline, and French), marketing only a fraction of these drugs, was selling $30 million worth of diet pills annually to diet-hungry American consumers.

Formula diet companies (the manufacturers of Metrecal, Sego, and the like) also do a big business. Their sales amounted to over $100 million (some estimates run up to $750 million) in the early 1960s when the formula diet craze was at its peak. Add to this the figures from a United States government survey indicating that $16,000 are spent *each minute* on various dietary devices and programs—or a staggering *$8 billion* over a year's time! Unless you're a stockholder in one of the companies in the weight loss business, it doesn't pay to be overweight. Obviously it can cost a great deal.

THE "CAUSES" OF BEING FAT

Fat, not weight, is the real menace to your health. You therefore need to watch out for obesity, or excessive fatness. In this section we ask the important question, how do people get fat? What causes the condition?

First of all, obesity is a *complex* condition, involving behavioral, physiological, glandular, metabolic, genetic, sociological, and economic factors. Exactly how these factors operate and how they interrelate are processes that are not well understood. Much more research is needed before they will be.

At one time only one factor was thought to be involved. For example, some considered obesity to be due to purely medical conditions such as an under-active thyroid gland, or genetic disposition; but these explanations apply to only a small number of cases.

Even when physical causes can be identified, however, their role is often secondary. For most people, *behavioral* factors seem to be the primary causes. The real culprit is the *energy balance* in your body, which is a balance between the energy you take in by eating and the energy you expend by physical activity. How you *behave* at the table and in your physical endeavors, therefore, has a direct bearing on how fat or slim you will be.

THE ENERGY BALANCE PROBLEM

The energy contained in food is measured in *calories.*[4] When you take in more food energy, or calories, than your body needs—i.e., for activities, growth, cell metabolism, digestion, respiration, a constant body temperature, and so on—the body converts the unused portion to fat. Since this conversion takes place at the rate of about 3,500 calories per pound of fat, for every *extra* 3,500 calories you consume, you become one pound fatter. The fat is then stored throughout the body and can be used for energy itself if an external food supply is not available.

The body's remarkable capacity to break down food and convert it to fat is a mixed blessing. In certain, usually primitive, circumstances, it can be very adaptive. For example, when people had to hunt for food there was no telling when and where they would see their next meal. At that time the extra fat on the body could always be used in an emergency, to sustain people until other food became available. But times have changed since we went hunting and gathering food. In today's

[4]Much more will be said about this in Chapter 5, when we talk about proper nutrition and the use of food exchange diets.

affluent, mechanized American society, food is in great supply for most people—no farther away, in fact, than the nearest restaurant or supermarket. If we eat too much and thus accumulate too much body fat, we usually *don't need* to use it later on. What was once adaptive then becomes maladaptive. As long as we keep eating more than we need, we'll just get fatter and fatter.

Energy balance, therefore, is an important concept, which will not only help you see how you have gained weight, but also how you can lose it.

Essentially three things can occur in your own energy balance. First, you can have a *positive energy balance,* in which the amount of food energy you consume is *greater* than what you expend. A positive energy balance can result either from eating too much food or from reductions in normal activity. Either way creates a positive balance of energy, and you're sure to gain weight. Remember, the unused food is being stored in your body as fat.

Second, you can have a *negative energy balance.* In this case the amount of energy you're expending, through exercise and normal metabolism, is greater than the food energy you're taking in. Like a positive energy balance, a negative balance can result in two ways: You can eat less or exercise more. Over a period of time with either solution, you'll start to lose weight and slim down. Ultimately a negative energy balance, in different ways and to various degrees, is what all diets seek to achieve. As you'll see later on, some of these ways are better for you than others.

Third, your energy balance can in fact, be *balanced.* In other words, the amount of energy you consume equals the amount of energy you expend. People who are able to *maintain* their weight at a constant level are doing nothing more than balancing their energy levels. Their eating habits give them all the energy they need to perform what they do, yet no more to gain weight nor less to lose it.

To take weight off, therefore, you need to create a negative energy balance by eating less and/or exercising more. To keep it off, you have to maintain the right energy balance. See Figure 1-1 for an illustrative summary of how the energy balance works.

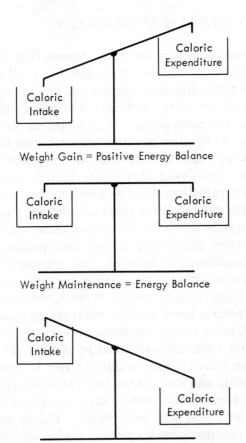

Weight Gain = Positive Energy Balance

Weight Maintenance = Energy Balance

Weight Loss = Negative Energy Balance

FIGURE 1-1

A positive energy balance can result from an increase in eating, a decrease in activity, or both. Conversely, a negative energy balance can result from an increase in activity, a decrease in eating, or both. The figure summarizes the relationship between energy balance and weight change.

Let's consider, in a little more detail, some of the factors that contribute to a positive energy balance or weight gain. As you'll see, there are quite a few of them.

REDUCED BASAL METABOLISM

Basal metabolism is the body process that produces the energy used to carry on such life functions as cell metabolism, body temperature, digestion, respiration, and heartbeat.

Measured at rest and at a comfortable external temperature, the basal energy needs of people vary with size, age, and sex. As for size, larger persons use more basal energy. Second, energy needs decline with age. Greatest in children because of their need for tissue-growth energy, basal metabolism is rapidly reduced as a person reaches full growth and eases off gradually throughout adulthood. If an adolescent of normal weight continues to eat the same amount of food when he reaches adulthood, he will gain weight because his metabolic requirement is reduced. This accounts, in part, for the expanding waistlines some people encounter in their early adulthood. Finally, sex is a factor. Women, for example, have a six or seven percent lower need for basal energy than men.

Though basal energy requirements vary along these lines, they also vary from one individual to another. The bodies of people of the same sex and weight can vary in how efficiently they digest food and store excess fat. These differences help to explain why some people seem to eat a lot and stay thin, while others eat little and still gain weight. The lower the basal metabolism requirements of a person, the less he or she needs to eat to maintain an energy balance and normal weight.

REDUCED PHYSICAL ACTIVITY

The technology, mechanization, and affluence of the twentieth century have at the same time increased our standard of living and *decreased* our physical activity. Machinery that saves physical activity in recreation also reduces our total energy expenditure, while power machinery cuts down substantially the physical energy expended at work. The gradual reduction in physical activity has, in part, caused the creeping expansion of modern man's waistline.

Let's take a look at some examples. A secretary who uses an electric rather than a manual typewriter uses 12 fewer calories (90 as opposed to 102) per hour. This may not seem like much of a difference. But multiplied by (20 hours per week × 50 weeks) per year, equals about 12,000 calories *not* used a year. Dividing by 3,500 calories to convert calories to pounds, 12,000 calories equals approximately 3.4 pounds per year—or over a ten-year period, approximately 34 pounds!

The car has also caused a major reduction in our energy expenditure. People drive to work, to school, to the store, to the theater, to the bank, to see friends, to church—almost everywhere. For example, a housewife drives two miles (round-trip), rather than walks, to the store twice a week. Over a year, she totals up 208 miles *not* walked. (Simply multiply 2 miles × 2 times a week times 52 weeks a year.) If approximately 88 calories are expended while walking a mile, 208 miles means 18,304 calories *not* expended a year. Converted to pounds, this represents 5.2 pounds gained per year or about 52 pounds over a ten-year period.

At home or at work the telephone extension has added inches to our waist while adding convenience to our lives. The American Telephone and Telegraph Company claims that an extension cord reduces walking by about 70 miles a year; it also reduces an individual's energy expenditure by about 6,160 calories per year (70 miles × 88 calories/mile). This many calories are equivalent to about 1.7 pounds of fat a year or about 17 pounds of fat in ten years. If extension phones are installed at home and at work at age twenty, and if everything else remains the same, a person could gain forty to fifty pounds by age fifty simply by not expending as much energy in walking to the phone.

Technology has also affected the level of physical activity

in some sports. Golf, a very popular participant sport, has been inundated with golf mobiles. Golfers are often encouraged at public courses and often required at private courses to ride golf carts rather than walk. Without a golf mobile on a typical golf course, a person would walk approximately 6 miles per 18 holes of golf, and approximately 1 mile with a golf mobile. A decrease of 5 miles × 88 calories/mile equals 440 calories *not* expended per 18 holes of golf. If a couple rode a golf mobile for 18 holes of golf each weekend, they would accumulate in one year about 22,880 unexpended calories (440 calories/18 holes of golf × 52 weekends). The calories, converted to pounds, come to about 6.5 pounds in one year, or about 65 pounds in ten years. Obviously, the only person who benefits is the owner of the golf shop that rents the powered carts.

A single physical activity by itself usually does not burn off many calories, but many different physical activities performed over days, weeks, and years can add up to many calories. In our examples, a person who uses an electric typewriter rather than a manual, who drives rather than walks to the nearby store, who uses extension telephones rather than one phone, who rides a golf mobile rather than walks at golf, *reduces* his or her energy expenditure by a staggering 68,496 calories per year! This is the equivalent of about 16.8 pounds per year, or the equivalent of about 168 pounds over ten years!

Jean Mayer, the noted Harvard nutritionist, has written, " . . . inactivity is the most important factor explaining the frequency of 'creeping' overweight in modern societies. Our body's regulation of food intake was just not designed for the highly mechanized sedentary conditions of modern life." [Mayer, 1969, p. 82]

Furthermore, the physical activity and basal metabolism levels of most adults decline as they grow older. Therefore any person who wants to *maintain* a healthy weight throughout life must *reduce* his or her food intake each year after reaching adulthood. This normal decline in energy needs, if not followed with a decrease in caloric intake, is often the cause of slow middle-age weight gains.

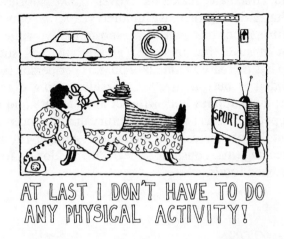

AT LAST I DON'T HAVE TO DO
ANY PHYSICAL ACTIVITY!

Courtesy of Dannon Milk Products. Used by permission.

AGRICULTURAL REVOLUTION AND AFFLUENCE

The agricultural revolution of the twentieth century has provided greater variety and abundance of nutritious food for a greater number of people than ever before in history. Yet there are millions of people who have not benefited from this revolution, and more work needs to be done to ensure that all people of the world have access to a healthy diet.

However, along with more nutritious food, there is also now available more high-fat, high-sugar, and high-carbohydrate food than ever before. Furthermore, the increase in the standard of living has made it possible for more people to buy these fatty, sugar-enriched foods than ever before—especially with the increasing use of quick, convenient, carry out, packaged foods which typically have a high calorie, fat, or sugar content. For example, a McDonald's hamburger, french fries, and chocolate shake have over 1,300 calories. In the United States during the past hundred years, the consumption of high-fiber foods has gone down substantially, while the consumption of sugar has increased greatly. In fact, sugar consumption has increased from 22.9 pounds per person in 1866 to 103 pounds per person in 1963.[5] Besides aiding digestion, a high-fiber diet supplies bulk without any calories and helps to reduce appetite.[6] Thus twentieth-century man has been decreasing his intake of low-calorie, high-fiber, hunger-filling foods and increasing his consumption of high-calorie, low-fiber, sugar-enriched foods.

FOOD ADVERTISEMENT AND PROMOTION

According to the U.S. Department of Commerce estimates, over $700 million were spent in the United States in 1973 on food and beverage advertisements. That money was spent to entice and condition us to eat more high-caloric, low-nutritious foods and beverages, such as carbonated drinks, beer, candy, pastries, and sugar coated cereals.

Promoters spend millions of dollars on advertisements to influence children's as well as adult's buying and eating habits. Recent studies on the influence of food advertisements on children have revealed that sixty to eighty percent of all children's commercials are for food, drink, and vitamin ads. The early conditioning of children's eating patterns probably influences them to eat larger portions of high-calorie, low-nutrition foods than they would otherwise.

Also the way food is promoted may deny people the opportunity to buy low-calorie foods. For example there is nothing

[5]*Agricultural Statistics* (United States Government Printing Office, 1973).

[6]Ruben, *Save Your Life Diet* (1975).

wrong with selling food from vending machines, but what concerns a growing number of health professionals is that most of the increasing amount of food sold in vending machines is junk food. Often nutritious, low-calorie foods are not stocked in vending machines.

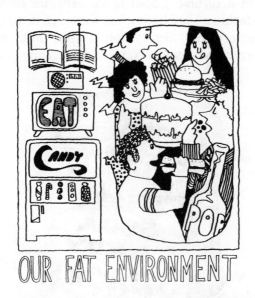

Courtesy of Dannon Milk Products. Used by permission.

Recently, a few educational institutions examined the influence of vending machines on their students. After evaluating the role of vending machines in increasing the intake of high-calorie, sugar-rich foods, the Dallas School Board passed the following regulation:[7]

The Board of Education believes that a student has the right to high quality nutrition and excellent health education. Vending machines in schools shall offer op-

[7]Dallas Independent School District, Administration Code 2480.5, Dallas, Texas, 1975.

timal choices to students and all foods and drinks sold in
vending machines shall be nutritious and selected for max-
imal appeal to students, excluding any foods or drinks
with a highly concentrated sugar base. Accessibility to
vending machines shall be controlled and shall not com-
pete with regular school lunch program or instruction.
. . . Machines shall be stocked with such items as fruit and
vegetable juices, dietary soft drinks, milk, nuts, seeds,
cheese products, crackers, fresh fruits, chips, etc.

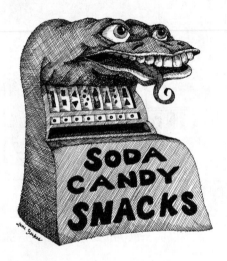

Vending machines invite us to eat foods that displace more nutritious ones.
Courtesy Smithsonian, *April, 1975.*

Because food is often promoted on the basis of appearance
and convenience and not on the basis of nutrition and calories,
clear and informative food labeling of nutritional value is often
neglected. Even if you have not already been heavily conditioned to buy high-calorie foods, and even if you find a variety
of foods to select from, you would have to be a nutritional expert
to figure out the caloric and nutrition values of the various
food choices.

Traditionally food labeling regulations in the United States have not required clear, simple labeling of the caloric value of food, so a person can easily determine how many calories he or she consumes. The U.S. Food and Drug Administration Labeling Act of 1975 requires the following information per serving: (1) serving size, (2) servings per container, (3) calories, (4) protein, (5) carbohydrates, (6) fat, and (7) percentages of U.S. Recommended Daily Allowances. The caloric content information of the food is especially convenient for the person who is trying to lose weight. Although these new regulations are an important step toward improving nutrition and weight management, nutrition labeling is voluntary for most foods. Only if a nutrient is added to the food or a nutritional claim made for it must the food include "nutrition information per serving."

The caloric content of cookies, candy bars, ice cream, beer, or soft drinks may not appear on these products. You may often buy these foods without knowing exactly how many calories are in them. The lack of complete food labeling, though not the primary cause of obesity, is certainly no help to you or to others in our society to lose or maintain a healthy weight.

Further research needs to be conducted to find out just how promoting high-calorie, low-nutrition foods increases obesity and other health problems in the modern world. At the moment, we do know that such food influences obesity.

SOCIOECONOMIC AND CULTURAL FACTORS

Obesity is a very democratic problem, affecting all segments of the population. Like the old saying about equality in a democracy, however, some people seem to be "more equal" than others.

Socioeconomic factors exert a powerful influence on the prevalence of obesity. Consider these findings and you'll see what we mean. Overweight problems are *six* times more common among women of lower social status than they are among higher-status women. Obesity is more prevalent among lower-class children than it is among children of the upper and middle classes. Another interesting piece of information is that social class is predictive of dieting. For example, among adult males increasing social status is associated with normal weight, and, generally, a disproportionately high number of people who are trying to lose weight come from upper socioeconomic groups.

The reasons for these findings are not entirely clear. Possible explanations include the effects of socioeconomic differences on food preferences, of income on the quality of food, of free time on exercise habits, and of cultural values on dietary behavior. In this latter case lower socioeconomic groups probably consume more inexpensive but higher calorie foods. They may also have fewer opportunities for vigorous exercise and come under less social pressure to lose weight.

Ethnic identity also influences the prevalence of obesity. For example, native (fourth generation) middle-class American women are *seven* times less likely to be obese than newly immigrated (first generation) Czech women of the same social class. Compared to first generation Hungarian, Puerto Rican, and Italian women, native American women are six times less likely to be overweight. Again, the most probable explanation for these findings has to do with differences in food preferences and eating habits. Ethnic groups that place a premium on starchy or fatty foods are more inclined to show a higher prevalence of obesity.

A Cautionary Note: While it's true that obesity is more common in some groups than others, don't assume that because you're in the "wrong" group you're stuck with your fat forever. At worst, these data suggest that it may be more difficult for some to lose weight than for others: Perhaps your family and friends are also overweight; perhaps you've been heavy for a long time; or maybe you'll have to make major changes in your usual way of shopping for food and preparing the family meals. Nevertheless, there's a big difference between a *difficult* task and an *impossible* task. Permanent weight loss is never impossible—no matter who you are—as long as you are willing to work at it.

FAMILY
AND PSYCHOLOGICAL FACTORS

Children learn much of their behavior by imitating their parents. If parents set bad examples, their children very likely will do the same, eventually. If, in addition, parents require their children to "eat all their food" and to "clean their plates," rewarding them when they comply and punishing them when they don't, their children will probably learn to eat to please others rather than to please their bodies. If parents handle stress and upset by eating, then it is also likely that their children will learn to do the same thing. Parents can have a tremendous influence in creating fat children or the disposition in children to become fat adults.

To be alive is to experience a myriad of feelings—feelings of joy and sadness, excitation and exhaustion, interest and boredom, calmness and anxiousness, companionship and loneliness. All people experience these feelings and more, and all people must learn to cope with negative as well as positive feelings. Unfortunately, the overweight person often eats to celebrate a victory and eats to soothe away the blues. Despite the many other ways to cope with life other than eating, the obese person often resorts to eating to cope with life. This "solution" quickly becomes a maladaptive response, resulting in becoming more overweight.

Social relationships may hinder weight loss or even encourage weight gain. For example our clinical research has shown us cases where spouses and friends who are overweight feel threatened or envious when the other one starts to lose weight. One, consciously or unconsciously, hinders or discourages the other from losing any more weight. We have even had cases where a spouse or friend encourages, tempts, and rewards the other person to become and stay overweight. For example, one spouse fattens up the other as a way to "prevent" the person from leaving or having an affair. Individuals have told us that if they fatten up their spouses enough they believe that the spouse will become so unattractive to others that they won't be able to leave them or have an affair—because no one else will have them.

These childhood, family, and psychological causes of obesity and what you can do about them are discussed in subsequent chapters.

*BIOLOGICAL
AND MEDICAL FACTORS*

All animals have genetically programmed appestats that control hunger and food intake—a very complicated system which is not fully understood. When energy reserves in the blood fall below a certain level, this mechanism triggers hunger sensations so that the animal eats. Each animal has a set point or thermo state for eating that controls how fat or thin the organism is.

The set point varies greatly between species, and can vary within a species. The set point can also be altered within a species by congenital defects, diseases, and early feeding patterns. For example, Prader Willi disease is a human congenital disorder that results in mental retardation and obesity. Cushing's syndrome is a tumor of the pituitary gland that gives rise to abnormal carbohydrate metabolism and results in obesity of the trunk and face. There are other congenital defects and diseases that can result in obesity, and certainly more will be discovered in the years ahead. However, present research indicates that these medical disorders account for only a *very small* percentage of obesity.

The set point appears also to be controlled, in part, by the number of fat cells. While the number of fat cells has been shown to be a function of heredity, Hirsch and his associates have conducted fascinating research indicating that early feeding patterns can also affect the number of fat cells.[8] Hirsch's research has found that baby rats who are overfed have more fat cells than baby rats who are not overfed. Once these fat cells are acquired in infancy they do not decrease in number as the animal grows or even when the animal loses weight. Rather, the number of cells remains about the same; only the size of the cells decreases.

The increase in the number of fat cells during infancy, it is therefore believed, raises the set point of the animal; consequently the animal needs to eat more to be "full," and thus maintains more body fat. Further, it is believed that even if the animal is put on a diet to reduce and loses weight, the disposition of the animal is to go back to its higher weight since the fat cells have a disposition to go back to their old, larger size.

Current research with humans, although still incomplete, suggests similar findings. Much is still not understood about the appestat and effects of early feeding, but the implications of this preliminary research are profound. Already the results have affected the thinking of pediatric health professionals regarding infant feeding. In the past a plump baby was considered a healthy baby. Most now believe that a plump baby will have a disposition to be a fat child or adult. Pediatricians and child development experts now recommend that infants *not* be overfed and a normal weight be maintained in individuals from birth to death. (See Chapter 13 for further information about child feeding problems.)

---

[8] J. Hirsch, J. L. Knittle, and L. B. Solans. Cell liped content and cell number in obese and non-obese human adipose tissue. *Journal of Clinical Investigation*, 1966, *45*, 1023.

In summary, current research indicates that medical disorders represent only a *tiny fraction* of the total overweight population. Of course when weight gain occurs suddenly and without apparent reason, it's always a good idea to check with your family doctor. He or she can rule out or tell you about possible glandular or other physical causes. But be prepared: Almost always *overweight comes from overeating,* not from medical causes. Clinging to the medical hypothesis ("I can't help it . . .") when no evidence for it exists is only fooling yourself—and doing yourself a disservice.

Also remember that even if you were heavy as a child or have a low metabolism, *you are not doomed to be permanently fat.* However, you may be susceptible to weight gain, and you will therefore have to be more careful about your weight than the next person. You can still have an optimistic viewpoint: After all, you can't change your medical history, but you can learn to control what you eat and what you do.

So far we've challenged a few prevalent misconceptions about obesity. For one, we pointed out that you can be obese without being overweight, and vice versa too. We have also shown why height-weight charts are not necessarily the best guide to determine your ideal weight. We have demonstrated the high costs of being overweight. And we have described the many causes of being fat, which for some of you, may have come as a surprise.

DEBUNKING SOME MYTHS
ABOUT DIETING

What are the facts about fad diets and pills? Hopefully the information in this section will put the problems of being overweight and of dieting into better perspective. If your last diet was a bust, you may see why it was—and how to avoid making past mistakes again.

MYTH #1: STARVATION
DIETS WORK

Starving yourself is one way to lose weight. But it's not a very good way for two major reasons. One is that fasting doesn't get at the heart of the overweight problem, which is teaching yourself to *live differently*—that is, changing your way of eating and exercising more. By necessity, starvation diets are short-term, a form of crisis intervention. Once the diet is over, your old habits take over again, and almost always you regain the weight you lost! The whole cycle (including the discomfort of starving yourself) must then repeat itself.

Starvation diets are ill advised also because they can often be hazardous to your health. Restricting your intake of certain food is one thing, but denying your body adequate nutrition is another. Your body needs a *balanced* diet of protein, fats, carbohydrates, vitamins, and minerals to function properly. Cutting out any one of them can upset your metabolism and make you feel uncomfortable or ill. Unbalancing your diet is a lot like denying your car oil, brake fluid, transmission fluid, or gasoline. When you do, the machinery doesn't work very well. The best type of diet, therefore, is one that is nutritionally sound and does not leave you feeling too hungry. With such a diet, you may have to wait a while longer to lose weight, but in the long run the wait is worth it.

MYTH #2: DIET PILLS ARE AN
EASY WAY TO LOSE WEIGHT

Many of us want workless wonders, effortless and fast. Because of advances in medicine and pharmacology, we have been led to believe that chemicals—pills—are *the* way to get rid of weight. While some pills can produce quick results (for example, aspirin for headache or antibiotics for bacterial infection), the value of diet pills has been vastly overrated. Those that are available without prescription contain very little medicine; they're practically useless from a medical standpoint. You may believe they're helping you (doctors call this a *placebo* effect), but chances are your belief is only superstitious. Check the instructions that accompany the pills the next time you set out to buy some. In most cases they'll tell you either *to restrict your intake of food or to lower the number of calories you consume,* in addition to taking the pills. Lowering your intake will take weight off, but the pills alone won't. Buying them is like throwing your money away.

Other types of prescription pills contain medicine, but they should be taken only under a *qualified* doctor's close supervision. Some pills, called "diuretics," alter your fluid retention system so that you excrete more water. They literally dry you out. People get hooked on diuretics because they seem to work so well and so easily, but the weight you lose is water weight, *not fat weight.* Although diuretics can be useful if you have a problem with water retention—a decision that should be made only by your physician—their sustained use can lead to such serious ailments as kidney damage.

Other diet pills that contain amphetamine are often called "pep pills" because they stimulate the body physically. This stimulation may enable you to burn off more calories and curb your appetite. But the usefulness of amphetamines is usually short-lived, about six weeks. After that period they may cease to have their original effect. In the meantime other uncomfortable side-effects can develop, such as insomnia, irritability, restlessness, tenseness, sweating, and a dry mouth. As pointed out earlier, there is also the real problem of physical and psychological addiction. Because these drugs are easily abused, their manufacture and sale are now regulated by federal and state officials.

MYTH #3: FAD DIET FANTASIES

Like old soldiers, fad diets never die. New ones just take their place. Over the years there have been countless miracle diets, crazes, and fads, each one promising a bit more than the others. Do any of these sound familiar? The Drinking Man's Diet, Zen Macrobiotic Diets, Metrecal Formula Diets, the Grapefruit Diet, the Rice Diet, the Ice-Cream and Bananas diet, the Amazing-New-You Diet, the No Willpower Diet, the diets of Drs. Stillman, Atkins, and Yudkin, *ad infinitum.* Each one of them has had its moment of glory and prosperity, and some are still quite popular today. Nevertheless, the fact that so many diets keep appearing probably says something about the effectiveness of them all.

Remember this about fad diets: Like starvation diets, they fail to get at the heart of the overweight problem—why you became overweight in the first place. The problem has to do with your living habits. Unless you change them permanently, any weight you lose from fad diets won't be any more permanent than weight loss through starvation diets.

Another problem with many of the fad diets is that they are *not* nutritionally sound. For example, you may have to eliminate carbohydrates entirely, while you eat all the saturated fats you want, as on Dr. Atkin's diet. Or, at the expense of a balanced diet, you may eat large quantities of recommended foods so unappealing that you probably won't want too much of them either—grapefruit, yogurt, rice, for example. Not only does this practice do little in the way of teaching you good eating habits—ones you can live with indefinitely—but, by restricting your diet to certain foods, it can upset your metabolism and harm your health.

Since it's impossible to go into all the health problems fad diets can cause, a good review on the subject can be found in Berland's *Rating the Diets,* published by *Consumer Reports.* You should just beware whenever a diet plan does not allow a well balanced menu. One writer described fad diets this way: "The main ingredient of these diets is baloney, and not the kind you eat."[9]

LOOKING AHEAD

According to the model we have presented, weight gain or fatness results from a positive energy balance. When we eat more than our bodies need, over a period of time our bodies do what they were designed to do, convert the excess food energy into fat.

Logically, something has to change before weight loss will occur. That something is *what we do*—our behavior. We have to either consume fewer calories (eat a little less than we did before) or burn off more calories by exercising more. Both ways produce a negative energy balance, which means your body will begin to use its own fat reserve for sustenance and you will lose fat weight. Furthermore, if you're able to maintain a better energy balance than you have before, you will have taken it off for good.

All of this seems simple and straightforward, and in a way it is. Certainly it is simpler than some of the high sounding weight loss schemes you've probably heard about before, but there is no inherent virtue in complex rhetoric. Simply stated, *this program for weight loss works*—slowly, yet permanently—and it does so without harming you.

On the other hand, permanent weight loss means perma-

[9]Knox, "Ten Common Misconceptions about Overweight and Dieting." *Better Homes and Gardens,* June 1972, p. 12.

nent habit change, and for most people that is *not* easy to achieve. A complex behavior like eating can be influenced by *psychological* factors (motivation, stress, boredom, anger), *biological* factors (metabolic requirements), *familial* factors (how others around us eat), and *cultural* factors (advertising, the availability of "junk" foods). All factors need to be taken into account if permanent changes are to occur. This plan will do that.

However, there are other things you should know about human behavior, some "principles of behavior." If you know how behavior works—conditions that influence how and what we do—you'll be in a much better position to help yourself. These principles, applied by you, can bring about better self-management, and so our next chapter is about the psychology of self-help.

2

The Psychology of Self-Help

Let's set the stage for the rest of the book by describing a way of looking at human behavior. This "way"—some people would call it a "theory" or "model" of behavior—has to do with behavioral self-control, an approach we call the *psychology of self-help*. But before we talk about self-help, we have to know what theories of behavior are all about—a somewhat broader issue. As you read along, you may see where some of your own ideas about behavior have come from.

THEORIES OF BEHAVIOR: A BRIEF OVERVIEW

Theories of behavior are by no means new, nor are they in short supply. For millennia people have tried to explain why they do certain things—the causes of their behavior. The question, "Why do we do the things we do?" dates back to antiquity, when Homer was writing of Odysseus and his adventures. That same question is no less challenging today. Although many different theories are available, none has been universally accepted. As you know, people are tremendously diverse and complex, leaving much room for disagreement.

All theories of behavior share a common purpose: to make sense of what people do. Despite a common purpose, not all theories are alike, nor are they of equal value. One of the many important differences among them has to do with *where* a theory encourages us to look for causes.

MENTALISTIC THEORIES

These theories emphasize the "mind" or other *mental* events as the causes of behavior. Have you ever been told to use your "willpower" to lose weight, or that losing weight really involves "mind over matter"? If so, your advisor(s) followed this type of theory. Their advice was based on the assumption[1] that mental events (or so-called *intrapsychic* events, because they are presumed to exist inside the psyche or mind) influence just about everything we do. Unfortunately, mentalistic theories rarely offer any *specific* prescriptions for behavior change. The unanswered question is, "How do you influence those mental causes?"

BIOLOGICAL THEORIES

These theories also look for the causes of behavior inside you, but in this case the causes are *biological,* not psychological. For example, some people believe either that overeating is a genetic problem or that the brain and the glands

[1]We use the word "assumption" because the existence of mental causes cannot be proven directly. They are *inferred* causes.

play a major role in determining our daily appetite. Weight loss programs that rely on shots (such as chorionic gonadotrophin), pills (amphetamines for example,), or surgery (like intestinal bypass operations) reflect this biological orientation—that is, to lose weight you must alter the underlying *biological* causes. Obviously, biological treatments require the close supervision of a qualified physician, because though they sometimes help, they are not without their associated risks and side-effects.

SUPERNATURAL THEORIES

A third—and from an historical standpoint, the oldest— type of theory attributes the causes of behavior to *supernatural* events, ethereal forces such as the spirit or soul. By definition, these forces cannot be observed. They transcend what people can notice or experience directly. Nevertheless, many people believe in their existence, and the power they supposedly wield. The statement "It's my fate to be fat" implies a belief in super- natural causes. Of course, this is not a very optimistic outlook, nor is it one that helps much when it comes to understanding and changing behavior.

The fact that these different theoretical viewpoints look for causes in different places has important practical and scien- tific implications, because some *potential* causes are more amenable to control than others. Many theories of behavior lack *practical utility,* encouraging us to look for causes we *can't con- trol*—causes that, in fact, may not even exist in some cases. On the other hand, if a theory tells us to look for causes we *can* control, it can be subjected to scientific scrutiny. Furthermore, *people can very likely learn to control events that influence them, in a way that they desire.* That's an important consideration when it comes to learning self-help or developing better self-control.

TOWARD A THEORY
OF BEHAVIORAL SELF-MANAGEMENT

In this book, we stress a *behavioral theory*.[2] More than anything else, this theory tells us that *learning* and the *environment* play vital roles in determining what we do.

The behavioral view is that the vast majority of our behaviors, including those we call self-control, are learned. We'll say more later on about *how* learning occurs, but it has to do with events and conditions around us—especially what the *consequences* of our actions are and what we *see others doing*. Just as we learn to talk, read, and engage in other complex activities, we can also learn to overeat or exercise too little. Further, learning is not an event that stops when we "grow up"; it is an ongoing process. We're never too old to learn new things or to do things differently. (Yes, even old dogs can learn new tricks, under the right conditions.)

Behaviorists assume that our environment exerts a powerful influence over what we do and when we do it. This term "environment" is interpreted broadly to include our *social* and *physical* surroundings outside as well as our ways of thinking or cognitions within us. When the environment remains relatively constant, we learn to behave in fairly consistent ways. But when the environment changes, very often our behavior changes too. To illustrate this point, consider the things you learned to do differently after you married, as you raised children, when the in-laws visited, or when you landed your first job. As the conditions changed, so did the things you did.

[2]For a more complete discussion of behavioral theory, you might want to consult B.F. Skinner's book, *About Behaviorism*.

And as conditions affect your behavior, your behavior can affect conditions. This two-way interplay is termed the *reciprocal influence* between behavior and the environment. Just as behavior is influenced by outer events acting on us (such as the reaction of others to the things we do), we also have the capability to act on the environment. We can, in effect, change our surroundings by our own actions, and in so doing we can arrange conditions to bring about desired changes in ourselves. The relationship between behavior and the environment is thus *interdependent;* that is, it works in two directions.

Essentially, this is what we mean by behavioral self-control. If we know how our behavior is influenced, we can create new and beneficial learning experiences for ourselves. We can arrange our environment, including what we do and whom we enlist for support, to make it possible for other desired changes to occur. As some writers have put it, the old Greek maxim, "Know thyself" can be paraphrased to mean "Know thy controlling influences."[3] If you know yours, self-help can become a very realistic possibility.

A PRESCRIPTION
FOR BETTER SELF-MANAGEMENT

You're probably saying, "Self-control is easier said than done. Enough talk—tell me what I can do!" What you can do is the goal of this section. Step by step we will spell out what behavioral self-control is all about and what you can *do* to achieve it.

The six steps to behavioral self-control are:

1. self-observing,
2. setting goals,

[3]See Thoresen and Mahoney, *Behavioral Self-Control.*

3. rearranging environments,
4. using graded practice,
5. using consequences properly, and
6. building commitment. We won't elaborate on any of these steps in great detail in this introductory chapter, but their presence will be felt throughout the book.

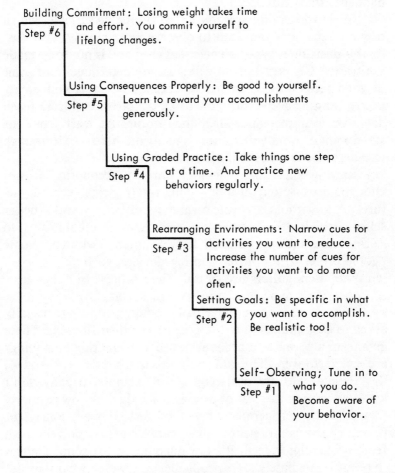

Building Commitment: Losing weight takes time and effort. You commit yourself to lifelong changes.
Step #6

Using Consequences Properly: Be good to yourself. Learn to reward your accomplishments generously.
Step #5

Using Graded Practice: Take things one step at a time. And practice new behaviors regularly.
Step #4

Rearranging Environments: Narrow cues for activities you want to reduce. Increase the number of cues for activities you want to do more often.
Step #3

Setting Goals: Be specific in what you want to accomplish. Be realistic too!
Step #2

Self-Observing; Tune in to what you do. Become aware of your behavior.
Step #1

FIGURE 2-1.
Six steps to better self-management.

1. SELF-OBSERVING

Concerned with "tuning in" to what you do, the purpose of self-observing is to increase your *awareness* of your own behavior. For example, how often do you snack or exercise each day? What happens before you do these things? And what happens afterwards?

In self-observing you must first decide *specifically* which of your behaviors you want to observe more closely. Obviously, this decision is based on personal need and is not to be made arbitrarily. Chapter 3 and 4 will help you determine what some of your needs may be. After the decision is made, you simply keep a running account of how often the behaviors occur (each day, for example) and when they occur. At least from the standpoint of what you do, that's really all there is to it (though in other ways self-observing is more involved).

Relying on rough memory for an accounting is not enough, because our memory alone rarely yields accurate pictures. And without accurate awareness of what you do, better self-control is very hard to achieve. A more reliable way to self-observe is to carry a small diary or notepad with you. Some people prefer to use little counting devices, such as the wrist-worn counters golfers use to tally their scores. In either case, self-observing involves accurate record-keeping.

In fact, as a part of self-observing, people are usually asked to keep graphs or written records of their findings. These give them a permanent account to use in evaluating how things are going. (More will be said about this in Chapters 3, 4, and 9.)

People who are overweight, for example, usually don't know how often they eat or exercise each day, or how regularly they raid the refrigerater when they feel stressed, lonely, or bored. Learning more about these habits can help prevent them from occurring; indeed, it's not uncommon for some changes to occur immediately after people begin to watch what they do. If they catch themselves doing things they don't like, they have a moment to stop and think—do they really *have* to do it? The stage is thus set for doing something else instead. On the other hand, observation of desired behavior (exercise, for example) may have the effect of increasing it for a while.

Self-observing is a helpful technique because it enables people to become more aware of themselves and their environment. The technique is usually *not sufficient* to produce lasting behavior change, but it's a step in the right direction.

One of the important results of self-observing is the continuous feedback it provides to the person, often telling him or her that things are getting better. This self-encouragement really keeps the desired changes going by serving as a commitment- or motivation-builder. But don't expect changes to occur indefinitely by self-observing alone. Other techniques are usually needed.

2. SETTING GOALS

Many of our behaviors are *goal-directed;* that is, we do things, like trying to lose weight, to achieve certain outcomes. These outcomes may be getting slimmer, looking nicer, or feeling better. Moreover, we want the outcomes to occur in certain ways—fast, for example. Setting goals takes into account the criteria or standards we use to evaluate our performance. Unclear or unrealistic goals and standards can make it hard to maintain the self-initiated changes we seek.

For example, people trying to lose weight often set exceedingly high goals for themselves. They may want to lose five, even ten pounds, in one week. Or they may vow never to eat sweets again! Unfortunately, what many of these people are doing (without knowing it) is setting themselves up for failure later on. Unless our goals are realistic and within reach, we rarely get to experience the good things that go with success. And without success, we find it easy to become discouraged, to put ourselves down, and to *give up* our noble efforts. The problem is not with people, however; it's with the nature of the goals they set.

Goals and standards therefore need to be set not too high and not too low—just high enough to keep you going and to make you feel good about your progress. As you'll see later on, one way to do this is to use both *long-range* and *intermediate* goals. (More will be said about realistic goal-setting in Chapter 4.)

3. REARRANGING ENVIRONMENTS

What we do does *not* occur in a vacuum. We learn to behave one way in certain situations and in other ways in different situations. You might say we learn to be *discriminating*—our behavior depends on the cues and events around us.

Consider any one thing you do. You'll find you don't do it *all* the time; instead, you're more likely to do it in certain situations than you are in others. For example, a behavior like saying "hello" usually occurs when we see someone we know or when we are greeted in a friendly way, but not when someone gets angry with us or when strangers pass us by. Similarly, a behavior like cigarette smoking is more likely to happen after eating a meal than when visiting the doctor's office. Other situations set the stage for eating—and overeating too.

All these examples have to do with the control of behavior exerted by *antecedent events;* that is, certain situational cues seem to encourage or prompt us to act in certain ways. Despite the fact that we do *not* behave like robots, and a behavior does not *have* to occur at any particular time, the likelihood of behaving in certain ways can be increased or decreased depending on the situation we're in.

What does this have to do with self-control, or more specifically, with weight loss? A great deal! Numerous studies have shown that overweight people are very responsive to situational cues when it comes to eating. In fact, *too many* external events seem to set the occasion for eating. Instead of eating when they feel true hunger, they eat when they get bored or upset, when they see or smell food, or whenever it's "mealtime."

Observing your own behavior will tell you if this is true of you. If it is, you don't have to sit by idly and continue in your old ways. *You can take some constructive action by rearranging your surroundings.* That is, you can eliminate many situational cues for eating and replace them with other cues. Even if certain cues *can't* be removed (such as watching TV or talking on the telephone), you can practice *non*-eating behaviors while watching TV or talking on the phone.

Though you'll see this self-control strategy used repeatedly in this book, for now a few brief examples will show you what we mean. Keep fattening (high-calorie) foods out of the house—or at least out of view; if they're not around, you'll be less tempted to eat them. Prepare smaller portions of food for yourself and your family; sometimes leftovers are a cue to keep on eating, even though you're no longer hungry. Have a list of friends or activities handy if you feel lonely, bored, or have nothing to do; instead of reaching for food, reach for them. Keep a graph of your daily weight and put it in a conspicuous spot—where you'll see it frequently; the graph serves as a constant and visible reminder to keep up with your diet.

4. USING GRADED PRACTICE

This *doesn't* mean to give yourself a letter grade (A, B, C . . .) for everything you do, as your teacher did in school. *Graded practice* means new habits are best acquired *gradually,* one step at a time.

Again, look at your own behavior to see what we mean. You don't do *now* what you did as an infant (sleeping, breathing, eating, and going to the bathroom don't count).

Your present skills and habits did not develop overnight; you learned them gradually, by doing them over and over again. After awhile they began to occur "naturally," with very little effort at all. Learning how to drive a car is another good example. Think about the many steps you went through to develop that skill, and how easy it has become since then.

The same approach works, therefore, when developing new eating and exercise habits. To get them going—and keep them going—takes time. But time alone is not enough: It's what you *do* with your time that counts. You have to practice.

Although overweight people share a common problem—too much fat on their bodies—they didn't all develop the problem in *exactly* the same way. The specific behaviors that contributed to it undoubtedly differ from one individual to another. The things they'll need to practice changing, therefore, will also vary.

In Chapters 3 and 4 you'll have a chance to assess your own eating and exercise habits to see where problems may exist. After pinpointing them, you can overcome them by practicing other new behaviors instead, a little at a time. You may have to slow down your eating, or avoid tempting situations that encourage you to eat. In other cases you may have to learn to say, "No thank you," to your hostess when second helpings are offered. Many of you may have to take up a new sport or hobby so that your exercise gradually increases. In all cases, developing new habits means practicing them. Learning may be a little hard at first, but if you take things gradually it should never be *too* hard.

5. USING CONSEQUENCES PROPERLY

Consequences, we know, play an important role in learning. What happens *after* we do something can make a big difference in whether we do it again.

In technical language, some consequences are called

reinforcers, because of their *effects* on our behavior. A reinforcer is a consequence that helps to *strengthen* behavior and make it happen more frequently. Basically there are two kinds of reinforcers:

1. A *positive reinforcer,* or a positive consequence, is something we'll work to obtain. A positive consequence strengthens the behavior it follows. For most people, positive reinforcers include such things as money, favorable recognition, praise, and the good feelings that accompany success. In many ways a positive reinforcer is like a reward, or something we value. Anything we work to earn is a positive reinforcer.

2. Other consequences are called *negative reinforcers,* or negative consequences. These are usually unpleasant events, things you try to escape from or avoid. An example of a negative consequence (at least for most people) is being nagged. When nagged, you usually do something to get away from the source, or sometimes nag back in hopes of stopping it. Whatever gets us away from something negative will be increased. Unfortunately, since eating often "gets us away" from negative feelings such as tiredness, anger, boredom, loneliness, or anxiousness, eating will be increased

Compared to negative reinforcers, positive reinforcers are a much more pleasant and effective way to go. And that's the approach we will take throughout this book. Arranging for good things to happen after the desired changes occur is a form of self- control.

Using positive reinforcers *properly,* however, is more complicated than it may appear at first glance. Arranging for nice things to happen is one thing, but how and when they should happen is another. Let's consider how positive consequences should be used for maximum effectiveness. We will discuss:

A. learning by successive approximations,
B. reinforcing our desired behaviors immediately *after* they occur, and
C. varying our positive reinforcers.

A. Successive Approximations.   Learning occurs best as you know now, when you take things one step at a time, and when you don't set your goals too high—especially when you're trying to develop new habits. Learning therefore occurs by *successive approximations.* This approach takes time, but eventually you develop new habits with a minimum of frustration or failure.

From the standpoint of using positive reinforcers effectively, taking small steps is important. We want you to use positive consequences as often as possible, for each bit of progress you make. If your goals are too high, however, good things won't have a chance to work. You'll never be able to satisfy yourself that you've earned them.

B. Immediate Positive Reinforcement.   Consequences work best when they *follow* desired behavior *immediately.* If they occur *before* the behavior takes place, they can backfire, helping to strengthen procrastination. If the delay between the behavior and the reward is too long, you might forget why you earned it in the first place, thus reducing its strengthening effect.

The importance of immediate reinforcement helps us understand why some people seem to *lack* self-control. Look at what's going on. For such behaviors as overeating, cigarette smoking, or overdrinking, two sets of important consequences are at work, one *immediate* and the other *longer-term.*

The immediate consequences are positive. For example, food usually tastes good and produces pleasant sensations in your body immediately after it is eaten. These positive consequences serve to keep the behavior going.

On the other hand, the longer-term consequences are negative—you may get fat, feel tired more often, and be restricted in your physical activities. But because these negative consequences are delayed, they are simply overshadowed by the more immediate, positive consequences. You act *as if* they weren't there at all. And in that kind of reinforcement much of the problem arises.

When you try to *break* old habits, like eating too much, the most important payoffs are long-range. There can be a considerable delay between cutting back on our eating and seeing results. The delay in the positive benefits makes self-control difficult.

How many times have you heard it said, "I'm so fat now, I'll never lose all the weight I want." Well, you can use other positive consequences, besides that *one* terminal goal, to keep your motivation high.

So most of us need help to bridge the gap between the behaviors we want to change and the long-range outcomes we seek. One way to obtain this help is to intentionally use *other* positive consequences, more *immediate* rewards to keep our motivation up and our commitment strong. If you don't use positive consequences immediately and frequently, your enthusiasm may quickly diminish. You'll stop doing what you started because the ultimate reward is simply too far away.

The same point applies when it comes to deciding what kinds of changes you should reinforce in yourself. As a general rule, *it's better to reinforce habit changes than it is weight loss per se.* Bad habits are the *cause* of the problem, and you must immediately reinforce the breaking of these habits. Weight loss will follow, but only if your eating and exercise behaviors change first.

C. Vary Positive Reinforcers. Hardly anything acts as a positive consequence all the time. If you get too much of a good thing, it can lose its positive value; you'll get tired of it. For this reason, *the greater the variety of positive consequences you have, the better.*

Positive reinforcers can be almost any thing, as long as *you find them to your liking.* That's a key point—you must find them pleasant. They may include *tangible* things such as a dress or book; *pleasant activities,* like going out on the town or to a show; *intangible* events, such as imagining a pleasant scene—maybe seeing yourself thinner. And don't be afraid to pat yourself on the back psychologically for the progress you've made ("Gee, I really did well yesterday by not eating too much"). Later on you'll have a chance to put together a list of events that might serve as good positive consequences for you.

Also, don't try to do it all by yourself. While you can give yourself positive consequences (so-called "self- reinforcement"), *you can also arrange things so that your friends and family help you out.* So enlist others to provide nice things when desired changes occur (so-called "external reinforcement"). As you know, an encouraging comment at the right time can be extremely helpful.

You can't however, always expect positive *social support* to happen naturally. You may have to ask for it or arrange for it in advance. Too often overweight people experience disappointment because this support doesn't happen. Unfortunately, others are not always sensitive to your progress. Upcoming chapters will deal with some suggestions on how to ask for the help of others. For now, just remember that the more positive consequences you have at your disposal—whether they come from you or others—the easier you will achieve self-control.

6. BUILDING COMMITMENT

Filling the prescription we've outlined in this section will probably mean making *major* changes in your present life style. There's no magic in self-control; nor is there any magic in learning how to help yourself. What's needed, however, is a strong sense of *commitment*—a decision to do things *differently* and to *keep at it.* Commitment takes a lot of patience, considerable effort, and much of your undivided attention, especially in the beginning.

This chapter was intended to generate a little commitment on your part. But since there can be no commitment without *direction,* our goal was to provide some direction too. You've seen that better self-control is possible and that you can achieve it.

The next chapter will help you assess your own commitment to lose weight *now*. It's an important chapter and we suggest that you read it carefully.

3

Are You Ready To Lose Weight?

To help you find out about yourself, we're going to ask you questions, some of which may seem difficult or take time to answer. For example, we'll ask you about your reasons for wanting to lose weight, and about the willingness of your friends to help you achieve this goal. In spite of their difficulty, however, we want you to pay close attention to each question and to be as complete and as candid in your answer as possible. It won't do any good to cheat or fool yourself, because honest self-observing is the first step forward permanent weight loss.

Altogether this chapter will take from one to three weeks to complete, but after you finish it you will know whether you are really ready to lose weight. You will also know what it takes to lose weight and keep it off. This understanding helps strengthen your commitment to succeed.

The primary question in this chapter is, "Are you ready to lose weight?" You will probably say, "Of course I am, otherwise I wouldn't be reading this book." We believe that you *want* to lose weight and encourage you to do so. However, before rushing into *another* diet, it's important that you carefully assess why you want to lose weight *now,* as well as some of the factors that may have contributed to unsuccessful weight loss efforts in the past. The better you understand these factors, the better you will be able to control them in the future.

The importance of carefully assessing your present readiness to lose weight cannot be overstated. Unless you are prepared to make a serious effort to change longstanding eating and exercise habits, you will probably fail to achieve the goals you set. Because we both want to avoid failure, we'll begin by discussing your own readiness to lose weight now.

WHY DO YOU WANT TO LOSE WEIGHT?

People want to lose weight for many different reasons: "My health will improve . . . I'll look better to myself and others . . . I'll be able to fit into my bikini this summer . . . I will have more energy . . . I'll feel better about myself . . . My spouse will quit nagging me about being fat . . . I'll have more friends . . . I'll be more attractive to the opposite sex . . . My job performance will improve . . . I'll get promoted at work . . . I'll be happier," and so on. While some of these reasons reflect short-term, as opposed to long-range, benefits of weight loss (such as wearing a bikini versus living longer), they all represent sources of motivation that can help to maintain proper eating and exercise habits. At this point you should begin to think carefully about your reasons for wanting to lose weight, together with the benefits you expect. Don't be discouraged if your reasons are not clear or if you feel unsure about them, because you may not have thought about them before. However, you must start thinking about them now in order to build the commitment that weight loss requires. So take time to write your reasons down in Table 3-1 before reading on.

Now look at your list and ask yourself, "If I lost weight, would I actually receive these benefits?" Some of your reasons for losing weight may be perfectly appropriate, while others may be entirely unrealistic. This is an important distinction. For example, when your weight returns to normal, you will probably be healthier, shapelier, maybe even sexier. However, losing weight will not automatically make you more popular with your friends or help you perform better on the job. Both of these goals may require changing other behaviors that are outside the realm of weight maintenance. Therefore go back and put a " + " by each statement you honestly think is an appropriate and achievable benefit of weight loss; then put a " – " by each statement you think is an unrealistic reason for losing weight. You are now developing a list of positive and realistic reasons for change—the first important step in helping yourself lose weight and keep it off.

As described in Chapter 2, many of our behaviors are maintained by the results or consequences they produce; that is, they are *reinforced* either when they are followed by positive experiences or when they take away or prevent something unpleasant. In analyzing obesity from this standpoint, it is meaningful to ask, "What are some of the consequences that maintain people's obesity?" Obviously there are many, and their precise nature varies from one person to the next.

For our immediate purposes we'll list only a few of these reinforcing consequences. See if they sound familiar.

—"I don't like to exercise nor do I have the time." Here the consequence is avoiding something unpleasant.

TABLE 3-1
Your Reasons for Losing Weight

Example: If I weighed 40 pounds less than I do now, I would look better.

1.

2.

3.

4.

5.

6.

7.

8.

9.

10.

—"I really enjoy rich pastries and desserts." Obviously certain foods are strong positive reinforcers.

—"I don't know what I'd do if I weren't munching on snacks." In this case eating acts as a negative reinforcer since it takes away something negative for us, perhaps reducing boredom and unstructured time.

—"Eating makes me feel better when I get angry or upset." Again, eating is negatively reinforced because it reduces emotional upset.

In the next examples see if you can identify possible reinforcers.

—"I enjoy going out to dinner with friends because it's the only chance we have to get together and chat."

—"If my weight were normal, I wouldn't have an excuse for not having many friends."

—"It's hard to say "no" to the in-laws after they've asked us over for dinner."

—"Sometimes I think my spouse really wants me to stay fat; after all, that's the way I was when he married me."

—"If I were normal weight, I wouldn't have anything to put myself down about."

—"There would be no excuses for not having a date."

These are just some of the consequences that can help to maintain excessive weight. Whether they are real or imaginary may not make a great deal of difference when it comes to changing eating behavior. In Table 3-2 list what you see as present sources of reinforcement for remaining overweight.

A comparison of Tables 3-1 and 3-2 will help you determine where your priorities lie. Do the weight loss benefits in Table 3-1 overshadow the reinforcers in 3-2? Can any of the benefits in Table 3-1 be used to immediately reinforce proper dieting behaviors? What about eliminating some of the pleasant consequences in Table 3-2 or making them happen *after* weight loss occurs. For example, could you use a special outing with friends (such as shopping for a new dress) as a reward for losing weight rather than an occasion to eat excessively? The proper use of reinforcing consequences was discussed in Chapter 2 and it will be discussed again in more detail later on.

WHAT IS YOUR WEIGHT GAIN
AND WEIGHT LOSS HISTORY?

Chances are your weight has vacillated in the past—you've put on pounds and even lost some at different points in your adult life. By considering your personal weight history, you may discover events that either led up to periods of weight gain or resulted in unsuccessful attempts to manage your weight. In this way you may also avoid encountering the same problems again.

People ordinarily gain weight when circumstances in their lives upset the normal balance between eating and exercise—between calories taken in and calories used. For example, you may have experienced a gradual weight gain as you grew older that resulted from engaging in less physical activity, even though you ate about the same. Weight gain may also happen suddenly. Sharp increases in weight can be caused by abrupt changes in normal eating and activity patterns when other things change, such as illness, marital conflicts, a move to a new location, pregnancy, and so on. Under these conditions you may have continued to gain weight even though the problem situation had passed. Once established, excessive eating and little or no exercising are difficult habits to break. *But they can be broken!*

So think about your physical, social, and psychological condition when these changes occurred. For example, did you

TABLE 3-2

**Sources of Reinforcement for Maintaining
Your Present Weight**

Example: Eating comforts me when I'm angry or upset.
1.
2.
3.
4.
5.
6.
7.
8.
9.
10.

first gain weight after a child was born, and then find it difficult to take it off because housework and child-rearing responsibilities seemed to prevent you from exercising as much as you would like? Did you gain weight after you stopped participating in a vigorous sport? (This often happens to persons after they graduate from school or reach middle age.) What about your physical and psychological state at these times? Did you put on pounds during an illness, or at a time in your life when you were under pressure at home or work? What was happening the last time you lost weight? Was a social event coming up when you wanted to look your best—or were your reasons more longlasting? Have you ever tried to lose weight before and failed, then felt that it was beyond your ability to do so? Any kind of failure can be a frustrating experience, which unfortunately may set the stage for further eating and even more unwanted weight.

When crash diets, fad diets, half-hearted diets, or miscellaneous "miracle" cures fail to produce lasting results (which they usually do), the consequence is negative—or at least not very encouraging. As failures accumulate, many people learn to avoid dieting altogether. After all, who wants to try and fail again? "What's the use, I know I'm hopelessly addicted to food" is the kind of self-talk that can easily become a self-fulfilling prophecy. All too commonly a person's inability to lose weight is perceived as a *personal failure* or a sign of moral weakness, rather than as the result of poor timing, inadequate social support, or (perhaps most often) improper dietary methods.

Eventually many people learn to excuse away their weight problems by calling them glandular, metabolic, or genetic. Have you ever heard, "I guess I'm the kind of person who can't lose weight. After all, my parents and grandparents are heavy too." Unfortunately, excuses do not solve problems; they only define them in different, usually unproductive, terms.

In Table 3–3 try to list (a) periods of significant weight gain in your life and the conditions that led to the weight gains,

(b) the nature of your attempts to lose weight, and (c) why you think you were unable to lose weight or keep it off.

At this point you might quickly review the events and conditions that may have contributed to your unsuccessful attempts at weight loss. What have you learned about yourself? Were there too many crash diets before? Were you *really* ready to change your eating and exercise habits permanently? Was your commitment to lose weight strong enough? Was your roommate or spouse helping out when you were trying to lose weight, or did he or she seem to cause more harm than good? Summarize your observations in the space provided on pages 61 and 62.

WILL IMPORTANT PEOPLE IN YOUR LIFE
HELP OR HINDER
YOUR EFFORTS TO LOSE WEIGHT?

Among the important people in your life are your spouse, relatives, friends, neighbors, and work colleagues. Relationships with these persons often involve advising and assisting one another. When you share any problem, your interactions with these persons may be hurtful as well as helpful. The issue of weight loss is no different. Some of your friends may want you to lose weight, and their efforts may be very helpful. Others may not understand how difficult it is for you to lose weight, hastily mumbling, "Just go on a diet"—perhaps with cigarettes in their hands, a habit they have been trying to break for years. Their *intentions* may be good, but their actions are little help. Some overweight friends may discourage dieting altogether because they could no longer participate in "fat" activities with you; they may even be envious of your achievements. In a few cases, a spouse or roommate may prefer you overweight, as a way of controlling you and protecting themselves. For example, spouses of obese clients have at times

TABLE 3-3
Weight Gain and Loss History

(a)Weight Gain when and why	(b) Weight Loss Program	(c) What Happened
First Time		
Second Time		
Third Time		

(If necessary, put additional times on a separate piece of paper.)

_____

_____

_____

_____

_____

_____

_____

_____

_____

_____

_____

_____

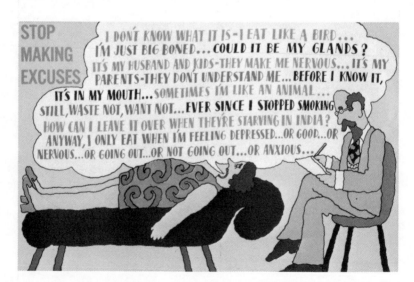

Courtesy of Dannon Milk Products. Used by permission.

admitted they wanted our clients to stay fat, because a weight loss would make them more attractive and more likely to engage in extramarital affairs. In other cases, both husband and wife subtly encouraged each other to overeat or mutually sabotaged their efforts to lose weight.

Think about the significant people in your life and how they interact with you—what they say and do. Which friends praise your efforts to diet, look forward to seeing you thinner, and don't tempt you with fattening foods? Conversely, which people reinforce excessive eating by reminding you of previous dieting failures, ridiculing your present weight loss efforts, offering you second helpings, or eating conspicuously in your presence? Trying to change your behavior without your friends *consistent support* is obviously a most difficult task. Since there are many ways for friends to help you lose weight, you must try to understand how important people in your life may aid or hinder your dieting efforts. Later in the book we'll make specific suggestions on how to enlist their positive support. For now simply consider the issue. Filling in Table 3-4 with the names of your "significant others" and how they might support or impede your weight control efforts may help you sort out your thoughts.

WHAT IS YOUR PRESENT PHYSICAL ACTIVITY LEVEL?

Research indicates that obesity is caused as much as physical inactivity as by overeating.[1] If you are going to lose weight and keep it off permanently, you need to make an honest and candid appraisal of your present activity level. (Later on, lessons will be included on how to use increased physical exercise to control your weight.)

[1]See Mayer (1968) for additional information on the relationship between physical activity and obesity.

TABLE 3-4
Significant Others List

Name	Relationship	Help	Hinder	How Will They Help or Hinder?
1.				
2.				
3.				
4.				
5.				

Physical activity means many things to different people. Our definition includes just about any activity that involves motor behavior. Routine chores, such as house cleaning, walking upstairs, and gardening, are just as valid as recreational activities, such as hiking, bicycling, tennis, and swimming. In Table 3-5 list your physical activities, how often and how long you do them, and how much you enjoy or dislike them.

WHAT ARE YOUR PRESENT EATING HABITS?

You might say that you already know what your eating habits are—awful! Without developing new eating habits you will probably put on excessive weight again, even if you succeed in losing it in the first place. That's why crash diets "crash."

TABLE 3–5

Physical Activity Review

Physical Activity	Minutes Spent Per Week in Activity	How Much You Enjoy or Dislike Activity
Example: *Tennis*	*90*	*enjoyed very much*
1.		
2.		
3.		
4.		
5.		
6.		
7.		
8.		
9.		
10.		

The first step toward changing your eating habits is to know what they are and what events influence them. Your present eating behaviors are probably guided by external cues in the environment as much as they are by internal hunger cues from your body. To illustrate this point, imagine yourself at a dinner party: After completing an extremely rich main dish your hostess asks, "Would you like some chocolate mousse for dessert? I made it just for this occasion." Your stomach says, "I'm full; no, I don't want anymore." But your social conscience says, "Eat it or you will appear ungrateful." As so often happens, we learn to respond to the *wrong* cues—those in our environment instead of in our bodies. We eat, but we are not hungry. Such behavior wouldn't be "wrong" if we usually did not respond to these social cues, and did not weigh too much. As another example, most people also encounter situations when they are upset or lonely, and some learn to comfort themselves by eating even though they are not physically hungry. Numerous other situations encourage eating by strong environmental cues. For example, dinner time, noontime, cocktail parties, holidays, vacations, watching TV are all often associated with ritualistic eating, or eating in the absence of internal hunger sensations.

Environmental food cues are so prevalent in our society that eating often becomes an unconscious routine. You therefore may be aware neither of how much you eat nor of the strong influence of environmental cues on your behavior. To get you more in touch with your eating behavior, maintain an eating record for one week (see Appendix A). In this diary you should record what, when, where, and how much you eat, as well as the feelings you experience while eating.

A sample data sheet (Table 3–6) shows how to record the quantity, type, and caloric value[2] of foods eaten, plus the situa-

[2]Although not essential, you may elect to calculate the number of calories you consume by looking up these values in the Food Calorie Chart at the back of the book. If some foods are not listed, a more detailed calorie counting book will probably include them.

TABLE 3–6

Sample Eating Record

Day: Friday
Date: August 8

Time Start/Stop	Quantity	Type	Calories	Situation: home, work, restaurant	People: alone, friends	Hunger and feelings
7:45–8:00 a.m.	1 cup 2 tbs	coffee with sugar	92	home	spouse	hungry, tired
10:30–10:45 a.m.	1 2 cups 2 tbs	sugared doughnut coffee with sugar	466 92	office	alone	starving
12:00–12:45 p.m.	1 med. 1 med. 1 glass	hamburger salad, no dress. iced tea, no sugar	350 75 1	office cafeteria	friends	moderately hungry, feeling relaxed
3:30–3:45 p.m.	2 2 1	candy bars cokes cookies	390 300 70	office	alone	not hungry, upset boss
6:00–7:00 p.m.	3 lg. pc. 1 cup 2 lg. serv. 3 med. pc. 1 cup 3 cups	bread creamed tomato soup mashed potatoes ham beets ice cream	180 188 170 800 60 520	home	family	not hungry, tired, upset, angry
8:30–11:00 p.m.	3 glasses 3 med. pc. 1 cup 3 cups	martini potato chips peanuts cookies	320 325 136 140	cocktail party	employees, friends	not hungry, tired, bored

Total 4465

tion, people, state of hunger, and feelings experienced while eating. This diary indicates that the person eats many high-caloric foods with little nutritional value. The person also eats in response to certain situational cues such as snacking at the office and eating when angry or bored.

You may be eager to start losing weight now, or embarrassed to record what you presently eat. But it is extremely important to monitor everything you eat first. For the next week at least, do *not* try to lose weight or alter your present eating habits. Eat as you do typically, *but be sure to record all pertinent information.* Be as honest and accurate as possible in recording the information. As noted before, deceiving yourself won't help. You must accept and realize this fact at every stage of this weight loss program. If nothing else, being honest with yourself builds a sense of commitment. And you'll need as much commitment as you can possibly generate to lose weight and keep it off.

WHAT IS YOUR PRESENT PHYSICAL HEALTH?

Before beginning this or any other dietary program, consulting your physician is always a good idea. A complete physical examination is also wise. Make sure that you are in good health and able to begin a long-term, gradual weight loss program. Tell your doctor about the program you are considering, discuss your weight loss goals, and try to gain his approval before you begin. Don't be discouraged, however, if he seems indifferent to your problem or skeptical about your ability— you can show him your success later on.

SUMMARIZING THE RESULTS OF
YOUR SELF-ASSESSMENT

In assessing your readiness to lose weight keep in mind that *right now* may not be the best time for you. Whether you decide to begin now or later is less critical than making a healthy decision that you can live with and that you can put into action. By all means, before beginning the program, you should feel a strong commitment to really succeed.

At this point, review your self-assessment by answering the following questions:

1. Did you complete all sections of this self-assessment and were your answers honest?   Yes____ No____

2. Do you have more positive and realistic reasons for losing weight than for remaining overweight?   Yes____ No____

3. Is your present commitment to lose weight stronger than past commitments?   Yes____ No____

4. Will important people in your life assist you to lose weight? Is their positive support a realistic possibility?
                                                       Yes____ No____

5. Are you willing to increase your physical activity in order to burn off calories and reduce hunger?   Yes____ No____

6. Are you willing to change your present eating habits?
                                                       Yes____ No____

7. Is your marital, home, and work situation stable enough to permit a long-term weight loss effort?   Yes____ No____

8. Are you willing to change inappropriate habits such as eating under stress or when bored?   Yes____ No____

9. Have you consulted with your physician about your present health and future weight loss goals?   Yes____ No____

10. Are you willing to commit yourself to a self-change pro-
    gram that will take time and effort?   Yes____ No____

    If you answered *yes* to all of these questions, you are ready
to undertake the weight loss program in this book. Skip the rest
of this chapter, turn to the next, and begin the treatment
phase.

    If, however, you could *not* answer *yes* to all of the ques-
tions, that's okay too. But roadblocks may be encountered
along the way, and these should be removed *now,* if at all possible, before beginning this or any other weight loss program. In
the meantime, you might consider the following suggestions:

1. Wait awhile until your marital, home, and work situations
   become more stable and conducive to permanent weight
   loss efforts.

2. Think about and discuss your own ambivalent feelings
   about wanting to lose weight with friends.

3. Talk with people you respect and ask them if they would be
   willing to help you lose weight.

4. If you feel your situation is personal, or that other problems will be difficult to resolve, you might consider seeking
   professional help. There are competent professionals in
   your area who offer marital, family, child, vocational,
   educational, and personal counseling. You can contact
   your family physician or a psychologist at a community
   mental health center for referral information.

4

Now Is The Time To Begin: Setting Realistic Goals and Rewarding Success

Let's quickly review the material we have covered up to now. In Chapter 1, our discussion of facts and myths about obesity should have cleared up any misconceptions you may have had, and put the problem of being overweight into better perspective. In Chapter 2 you were introduced to the topic of behavioral self-management, an approach we call the *psychology of self-help.* In the last chapter you took an important first step toward beginning a weight loss program: You assessed your readiness to lose weight and answered a series of questions to start you toward that goal. Assuming your readiness and commitment are high, *now is the time to begin.*

If your spouse, a friend, or friends also want to lose weight, then skip ahead and read Chapter 12, "Weight Loss for Two or More." Discuss with them whether they would like to lose weight with you. Suggest that they also read this book and see if they want to lose weight now. If they do *not* want to lose weight with you, then simply continue on your own. If they do want to lose weight with you, consider carefully the ideas in Chapter 12 about *contracting* for habit changes. Use these ideas about contracting with others as you progress through this and later lessons.

In the remaining chapters, therefore, we will talk about how *you* can permanently change your eating, exercise, and life style habits. There is no way around permanent changes of habit; successful weight loss requires them. As much as we would like you to sit back, relax, and let the wonders of modern science take the pounds off for you, there are no effortless ways to lose weight and keep it lost. To suggest otherwise would only create misleading expectations, something we both want to avoid. But even though there are no genuinely easy ways to lose weight, *you* can do it slowly yet surely. That's important. By trying hard, by being patient with yourself, and by sticking to your commitment, you will be on your way to kicking the overweight habit for good.

The next six chapters are organized around specific lessons:

1. setting realistic goals and rewarding success;
2. decreasing caloric intake by dieting;
3. increasing energy expenditure by physical activity;
4. enlisting positive support from family and friends;
5. finding better ways to manage food; and
6. learning to handle your feelings and to solve problems without eating.

The format of all the lessons is first to help you identify current "problem" behaviors, then to select alternative behaviors as substitutes. As you do this, you will be *developing your own program* for change.

Although each chapter is designed to take from one to four weeks to complete, some of them may take a little longer. Rather than set a rigid schedule for you, we feel you should master each lesson at your own pace. Go on to the next chapter only when you think you are ready. There is no need to feel rushed. Permanently breaking old habits takes time.

You will soon see that each chapter (or lesson) requires you to be an *active participant,* to be both student and teacher. Acquiring and perfecting new habits is not a spectator sport: You can't just buy a ticket, sit in the stands, and casually watch the pounds leave the field. Losing weight is an active process, one that requires self-study and systematic practice. By following the lessons closely, you will become more aware of your behavior and learn to control your weight safely and effectively, which is the long-range goal you want to achieve.

SETTING REALISTIC GOALS IS IMPORTANT

We tend to judge ourselves by the goals we set. When we reach our goals, we experience a sense of mastery. Psychologically we pat ourselves on the back. We feel good. These positive feelings reinforce our efforts and encourage us to continue the activities that produced the good feelings. Conversely, when we fall short of our goals we sometimes experience bad feelings—frustration, self-doubt, anger, pity, sadness, to name but a few. Since these feelings are unpleasant, we usually avoid the behaviors that brought them about. We may even conclude that the goals we seek are forever beyond our reach. One way or the other, the goals we set influence our ability not only to attain them but to sustain goal-seeking behaviors as well. The process of setting goals, therefore, deserves close attention.

Overweight people who set unrealistically *high* weight loss goals are almost certainly doomed to fail from the start.[1] Consider, for example, a 38-year-old woman who wants to lose fifty pounds in the two months left before her twenty-year high school reunion party. While she might imagine that being the same weight when she last attended high school would be great, she must lose almost a pound a day. Her goal is unreasonable since she's very unlikely to reach it. When she discovers this (the hard way), she will probably feel frustrated and angry at herself. Since a common way to seek relief from such negative feelings is through "binge" eating, setting unrealistic goals can backfire in the long run, to *increase* the very activities we intend to eliminate.

What is a realistic goal? Unfortunately no precise answer can be given, because absolute rules do not exist. We believe that realistic goals should be based on an accurate assessment of each person's behavioral strengths and weaknesses. Also important are the kind of environmental pressures acting upon the person, as well as the motivational factors—namely, how much conscious effort the person is willing to spend to attain the goals he or she sets. The more completely we assess these issues, the better we are able to set attainable goals.

Because such long-term goals as permanent changes in eating, exercise, and life styles habits are so far off in the future, more immediate goals are needed to sustain our efforts and to keep us on the right track. We can call these *short-term,* or *intermediate goals.* Short-term goals allow us to measure progress over shorter periods of time, and to call attention to success regularly as these short-term goals are reached. For example, a person's long-term weight loss goal might be to lose 20 pounds during the next four months, then to maintain the loss indefinitely. The same person's short-term goals may include: (1) attaining weekly weight loss goals of from one to two pounds

[1]A study by Chapman (1976) showed that realistic goal-setting was a very important factor among those who lost weight successfully.

per week, (2) gradually increasing exercise levels from one week to the next, (3) correcting a specific eating habit, and so forth. A *combination* of *realistic short- and long-term goals* help to put weight loss efforts into better perspective, by providing a yardstick to measure progress each step of the way.

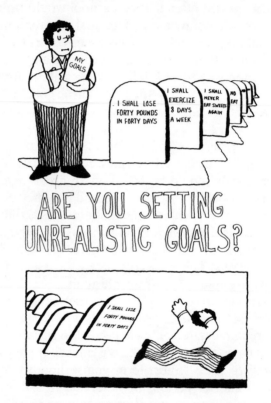

Courtesy of Dannon Milk Products. Used by permission.

This continuous feedback is extremely important because it maintains our commitment when other rewards are slow in coming. By using several short-term goals we prevent or guard against getting too discouraged. For example, we might fall short in losing weight for the week, but succeed in changing food choices and in doing some physical exercise each day.

AN OPTIMAL WEIGHT FOR YOU.

Your optimal weight is determined by several different considerations. Tables 4-1 and 4-2 show weight ranges considered to be healthy for adults of varying sizes and ages. Weight *ranges* are presented, instead of specific weights, because persons differ in physique, bone structure, muscle tone, and the weight they feel most comfortable at.

TABLE 4-1
Desirable Weights for Men
(Ages 25 and Over)*

Height (without shoes)		Weight in Pounds According to Frame (in Indoor Clothing)		
Feet	Inches	Small Frame	Medium Frame	Large Frame
5	1	112–120	118–129	126–141
5	2	115–123	121–133	129–144
5	3	118–126	124–136	132–148
5	4	121–129	127–139	135–152
5	5	124–133	130–143	138–156
5	6	128–137	134–147	142–161
5	7	132–141	138–152	147–166
5	8	136–145	142–156	151–170
5	9	140–150	146–160	155–174
5	10	144–154	150–165	159–179
5	11	148–158	154–170	164–184
6	0	152–162	158–175	168–189
6	1	156–167	162–180	173–194
6	2	160–171	167–185	178–199
6	3	164–175	172–190	182–204

*Courtesy of the Metropolitan Life Insurance Company, New York, N.Y. Derived from data of the 1959 Build and Blood Pressure Study, Society of Actuaries.

In selecting your long-range weight goal, we suggest that you set it at the upper end of the "medium frame" range for your height. When you reach that goal, see how it feels. If you want to lose more weight, you can reset your goal at that time. If you're already in a weight range for your height in the

TABLE 4-2

Desirable Weights for Women

(Ages 25 and Over)*

Height (without shoes)		Weight in Pounds According to Frame (in Indoor Clothing)		
Feet	*Inches*	*Small Frame*	*Medium Frame*	*Large Frame*
4	8	92- 98	96-107	104-119
4	9	94-101	98-110	106-122
4	10	96-104	101-113	109-125
4	11	99-107	104-116	112-128
5	0	102-110	107-119	115-131
5	1	105-113	110-122	118-134
5	2	108-116	113-126	121-138
5	3	111-119	116-130	125-142
5	4	114-123	120-135	129-146
5	5	118-127	124-139	133-150
5	6	122-131	128-143	137-154
5	7	126-135	132-147	141-158
5	8	130-140	136-151	145-163
5	9	134-144	140-155	149-168
5	10	138-148	144-159	153-173

*Note: for girls between 18 and 25, subtract one pound for each year under 25. Courtesy of the Metropolitan Life Insurance Company, New York, N.Y. Derived from data of the 1959 Build and Blood Pressue Study, Society of Actuaries.

"medium frame" category, but still feel heavy, select a weight goal in the "small frame" category.

In addition to using an ideal weight table, you can also use the old pinch test (see Chapter 1). This test, you'll recall, consists of gently pinching the area under your arm (triceps) or the area around your waist. Flabbiness or softness in either area indicates excessive fat, and you may want to exercise more to firm up the muscles as well as just lose weight.

Let's illustrate how someone might determine his or her best weight. For example, a woman who is 5'5" and weighs 195 pounds should probably set her initial long-term goal at 139 pounds, the weight suggested at the upper end of a medium frame for a woman of her height. After she reaches her goal of 139 pounds, she can give herself the pinch test, evaluate how she feels, and set a lower goal if she still feels overweight. This sensible approach to goal-setting leads to success and self-satisfaction in the long run. Setting a weight loss goal appropriate only for a sleek fashion model or race horse jockey—unless that is what you want to be—is simply unrealistic.

BE GOOD TO YOURSELF: LEARN TO
REWARD SUCCESSES

As described in Chapter 2 one way to increase behavior is to use rewarding consequences. The idea of rewarding is used in the spirit of stimulating and encouraging. When a desired behavior occurs, it should be followed by something nice. If it does not occur, then encouraging events are best withheld.

In Chapter 7 you will be taught to ask other people to encourage you for making successful changes in your eating and exercise habits. But no matter how helpful others may be, they will not be with you continuously. They cannot always be counted on to reward you immediately after desired changes take place. There is only one person who can do this—*you*.

You might assume that rewarding yourself is simple and really unnecessary. For example, all you do is wait until you have lost about ten pounds, then treat yourself by going out to dinner. Right? Wrong! The appropriate use of self-reward is not that easy; it is a skill that must be learned.

What are the problems with the way self-reward was used in the example above? To begin with, the person did not really know how much weight he or she had lost; an estimate of "about ten pounds" is not the same as knowing for sure that rewards have been properly earned. Second, the weight loss goal was not specified very well; in addition, it was unrealistically high. This person, unfortunately, is learning only to be arbitrary and miserly with himself, and neither of these attributes are very helpful when it comes to producing desired behavior change. Finally, the chosen reward was food, when other rewards might have served equally well. You'll find a major cultural problem is that food has become the remedy for all our ills as well as the reward for all our triumphs. Not using food as a reward is difficult but possible. Even though food is often used as a reward by some people, it is obviously the kind of reward you want to avoid.

What are some other rewards? Basically, a reward can be almost anything, if you find it pleasurable and can give it to yourself *after* you have succeeded at some weight control task. Possible rewards include doing *preferred activities,* such as hobbies, shopping for clothes, talking to friends, taking in a movie, listening to records, and so on. They may also be *positive self-statements,* nice things you can say to yourself: for example, "I feel proud of myself . . . I knew I could do it . . . I handled that situation very well." Another class of rewards is *symbolic events,* such as imagining—or getting a mental picture of—how much better you will look when you reach your ultimate weight loss goal. Whether rewards are tangible, spoken, or imagined may not make a great deal of difference when it comes to motivating behavior. As long as they make you feel good, use them frequently. Frequent use will strengthen your commitment and encourage your new behaviors as well.

Essentially, then, rewards are highly individualized: Whatever is *personally satisfying* can be a reward for you. Table 4–3 is a "reward menu" generated by one person. In it are listed various rewards of an *overt* and *covert* (verbal/mental) nature. After looking the table over, use Table 4–4 to put together your own list of rewards. The instructions for completing the table are quite simple: In list "A, Rewarding Overt Activities," write down some enjoyable activities or things you can treat yourself to when desired changes take place. In list "B, Rewarding Covert Activities," write down a few positive self-statements or pleasant images that might also serve as self-administered rewards. Try to be as specific as you can, and remember that these consequences need be pleasant only for you. Whether others would find them enjoyable is not important.

TABLE 4–3

Louise's Reward Menu: A Case Illustration

A. Rewarding Overt Activities
1. *Going to a movie with husband* 11. *Taking a long hot bath.*
2. *Listening to music.* 12. *Taking a morning nap.*
3. *Reading.* 13. *Visiting friends.*
4. *Doing needlework.* 14.
5. *Playing golf.* 15.
6. *Bicycling.* 16.
7. *Calling a friend.* 17.
8. *Watching television.* 18.
9. *Shopping for clothes.* 19.
10. *Writing personal letters.* 20.

B. Rewarding Covert Activities
1. *Thinking about the new me.*
2. *Imagining relaxing in my favorite chair.*
3. *Saying to myself "I exercised; I'm doing well."*
4. *Recalling my past accomplishments.*
5. *Saying to myself, "I'm proud of what I did ..."*
6. *Thinking how great it will be to wear a smaller dress.*
7. *Imagining getting in and out of the car more easily.*
8.
9.
10.

Though ultimately you want to become thinner, healthier, and happier, you can maintain your efforts and make them more enjoyable by rewarding yourself now, immediately after relevant weight management behaviors are performed. After

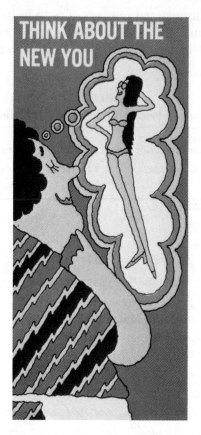

Courtesy of Dannon Milk Products. Used by permission.

every lesson you complete, try rewarding yourself by some
positive self-talk ("I'm proud of myself"), then select an activity from list A or B and enjoy yourself for having done a good
job. You might also reward yourself for refraining from snacking when the urge is great, or for a small loss in weight over
your previous day's amount. Always keep in mind the notion of
the selective application of rewards: *If* desired changes occur,
then do something nice for yourself. Rewarding events work
best when they *follow* the behavior we seek to change and when
they are *not* available to us at other times.

TABLE 4-4
Your Reward Menu

A. Rewarding Overt Activities

1.	11.
2.	12.
3.	13.
4.	14.
5.	15.
6.	16.
7.	17.
8.	18.
9.	19.
10.	20.

B. Rewarding Covert Activities

1.

2.

3.

4.

5.

6.

7.

8.

9.

10.

WAYS TO HANDLE TEMPORARY
SETBACKS AND DISCOURAGEMENT

No matter how well you plan ahead, or how hard you work at losing weight, there will probably be times when you fail to meet some of your short-term goals. Perhaps you will reach a temporary plateau because the goal itself is too high, or you won't follow your dietary plan completely. Typically, you will feel discouraged, put yourself down, then eat to "soothe your blues." You might tell yourself something like, "I've blown it. What's the use? I may as well eat all I want now. I'll begin the darn diet later on." In the meantime you will gain back all the weight you lost, perhaps even more.

There are better ways to handle failure. First, *you never fail:* You only make mistakes that teach you valuable things. Use errors to carefully consider what went wrong; they are sources of important information. Ask yourself, "Why didn't I achieve the goal I set?" Then try to come up with some answers. Maybe you failed to keep track of everything you ate. Or perhaps you set an unrealistically high goal for the week. (Thinking small is not really un-American, you know.) Maybe you were too stingy or forgot to reward yourself for small prior successes. These are all possible factors that can slow your progress. They are also correctable!

Try to discover what produced your setback and what you can do, beginning with your next meal, to change the situation. If you have regulated your eating Monday through Friday, but lapse on the weekend, have you blown it for the whole week? Of course not! You have succeeded for five of the seven days. You should feel good about that and reward yourself accordingly. After all, it's probably a big improvement over what you used to do.

5

Taking In Calories and Diets

To lose weight permanently you must permanently change your eating and physical activity habits, and no special "crash" diet will produce such long-lasting changes. Even though many people have lost weight by fasting or going on a special grapefruit or prune diet, few are willing to remain on such a diet for the rest of their lives. Thus, after they lose weight on a crash diet, these people usually resume their *old* eating habits—the very behaviors that caused the weight problem in the first place! For effective weight control, therefore, people must develop eating patterns that they can live with comfortably for the rest of their lives and still maintain a desirable weight!

Crash starvation diets always crash; they have no lasting value. They fail because they don't get at the heart of the problem—how you eat when you are *not* dieting. Rather, you should attempt to find a reasonable balance of nutritious, delicious, low-calorie foods that can be maintained for life.

You must learn to break the old habit patterns of eating snacks while preparing meals, eating while watching television, eating everything placed before you at mealtime, and so on.

Before planning your diet, let's first review some basic facts about nutrition which can be helpful to you in your weight loss attempt. Then we will present a common sense diet and a more comprehensive food exchange diet. You will then be guided in selecting and implementing a low-calorie diet that you can live with.[1]

BASIC FACTS ABOUT NUTRITION

Our body uses food as a source of fuel to provide energy to keep it running and as a source of nutrients to continually repair and maintain all tissues. Almost all foods can serve as fuel for energy, but no single food provides all the essential nutrients. Consequently we need a *balanced diet* of different foods. Most foods are a mixture of protein, carbohydrate, and fat along with varying amounts of vitamins and minerals. (You can now see why some crash diets may even be unhealthy for you because they don't provide a balanced diet.)

PROTEINS

Essential for the growth, metabolism, healing, and upkeep of our bodies, there are many different types of protein. However, all proteins are formed from the same twenty chemical components called amino acids. Like letters in an alphabet, these amino acids can be combined in a number of ways, each combination constituting a different protein; some very large protein molecules consist of hundreds of amino acids.

[1]Thanks are extended to Donna M. Watson, Registered Dietician, for her suggestions on the sections dealing with nutrition and food exchange diets.

While our bodies can convert some amino acids into others, eight essential aminos cannot be synthesized by us, and we must therefore get them from the food we eat. Basic sources of protein are dairy products, meats, poultry, seafood, legumes (beans, peas, peanuts), nuts, and seeds. Our diet should contain a variety of these protein-rich foods.

CARBOHYDRATES

The chief function of carbohydrate is to supply sugar (or glucose) as fuel for the brain and muscle tissue.

By limiting our intake of carbohydrates, and total caloric intake, we force our bodies to draw on stored fat and sometimes protein for our fuel requirements. But some carbohydrate is required in a balanced diet, because the lack of it causes several problems. For one, the body has to convert protein into sugar needed by the brain. Low-carbohydrate/high-fat diets may not provide enough carbohydrates to adequately metabolize dietary fat, which can lead to unhealthy side effects. Another problem with unbalanced "starvation" diets is that it causes our bodies to use lean body mass to meet our glucose needs as fuel for the brain and body.

In contrast, a moderate, balanced diet results in a regular weight loss of one to two pounds per week and avoids unhealthy side effects. Grains such as wheat, starches, vegetables, and sugar are common sources of carbohydrates. Any excess carbohydrate in our daily diet is converted to fat and stored in the body.

FATS

The most concentrated form of energy, fats serve primarily as a fuel storage material. A few fatty acids are considered essential and cannot be manufactured in the body.

There are both animal and vegetable fats. Common animal fats are butter, bacon fat, and the cream in milk; common vegetable fats are soybean oil, corn oil, olive oil, and peanut oil. Research indicates that high-cholesterol and high-saturated-fat diets not only lead to extra pounds but also increase the risk of heart disease. In general, it is a good idea to reduce your intake of fats, particularly the saturated fats found in most animal products.

VITAMINS, MINERALS AND WATER

Though your body must have these elements and compounds to function normally, it cannot manufacture them. If they're not in your diet, your body will therefore be deficient. Vitamin deficiencies can lead to such diseases as beriberi, scurvy, pellagra, rickets. The lack of minerals can affect our metabolism as well as the formation of bones and teeth. A mineral deficiency of iodine, for example, can lead to diseases such as simple goiter. Water is also essential for natural body functioning; most of us could not survive for more than a few days without water, though we can survive much longer without food. Table 5-1 lists the essential vitamins and minerals as well as foods rich in these nutrients.

A COMMON SENSE DIET

According to our energy balance model, to lose weight you need to reduce your caloric intake. Some people already know about calories and, in general, they have a balanced diet. Their problem is reducing their total caloric intake of food. These people may also be aware of particular problem areas, such as taking second helpings or eating continuously while watching

TABLE 5-1

Vitamins, Minerals and Their Food Sources

Nutrient	Common Food Sources
Vitamins	
Vitamin A	butter, eggs, liver, milk, vegetables
Vitamin B₁ (Thiamine)	cereals, beans, meats, nuts
B₂ (Riboflavin)	cheese, eggs, green leafy vegetables, liver, milk
B₆ (Pyridoxine)	cereals, liver, meats, wheat germ
B₁₂ (Cobalamin)	eggs, dairy products, meats
Niacin	beans, whole grain cereals, liver, meats
Folic Acid	beans, whole grain cereals, liver, peas, green leafy vegetables
Vitamin C (Ascorbic Acid)	citrus fruits, broccoli, melons, strawberries, tomatoes, green leafy vegetables
Vitamin D	fish liver oils, milk fortified with vitamin D, sunlight
Vitamin E	whole grain cereals, eggs, wheat germ, vegetable oils, margarine
Vitamin K	egg yolk, liver, soybean oil, green leafy vegetables
*Minerals**	
Calcium	dairy products, green leafy vegetables
Iodine	iodized salt, vegetables, seafoods
Iron	dried fruits, meat, green leafy vegetables, enriched bread and cereals
Magnesium	beans, whole grain cereals, nuts, peas, green leafy vegetables
Phosphorus	dairy products, eggs, meat

*These are the most common minerals. If your diet provides sufficient quantities of these minerals, other essential minerals will also be provided.

television. These people often know what they need to do and can start reducing their caloric intake without following a structured diet. If you think you are one of these people and can work better without a structured diet, then follow the list of general guidelines for dieting and reduce your caloric intake for about three to four weeks. After that period, evaluate whether your eating habits and weight have changed. If they have, reward yourself and continue doing what works best for you. If you still haven't changed your eating habits, or if you still are not getting a balanced diet, or if you are not losing weight, then we strongly recommend that you read and follow the next section on a food exchange diet.

A FEW GUIDELINES ABOUT DIETING

1. Your daily diet should be a well-balanced one, high in protein and low in carbohydrates and fats. However, do *not* eliminate all carbohydrates and fats.

2. Avoid crash starvation diets.

3. Substitute lower-calorie foods for your present ones. Become familiar with the "calorie cost" of different food categories.

4. Make room for an occasional snack or sweet by cutting down elsewhere in your food intake. Do not forbid yourself certain foods—this only makes them more tempting. It also increases the chances that you will simply give up once you have "blown your diet" by eating "a forbidden fruit."

5. Include a variety of foods in your diet, and avoid rigid, limited menus.

6. Don't skip meals. Avoiding overeating is easier if you are not overhungry. In particular, don't skip breakfast since it is the first meal after an overnight fast. Studies have shown that, when breakfast is missed, performance decreases while hunger increases.

7. If you find that you are hungry before mealtime, control your appetite by drinking a glass of water or juice with a tablespoon of bran about a half hour before mealtime. The bran helps give you a full feeling, reduces hunger, and adds a small amount of natural fiber to your diet.[2]

[2]The book *Save Your Life Diet* by David Ruben discusses the advantages of including bran in your diet to lose weight as well as to add more natural fiber to your diet.

A FOOD EXCHANGE DIET

Most overweight people do *not* eat a balanced diet; they are *not* aware of their eating patterns, or they need a *more* structured diet to help them lose weight. If you think you are one of these people, then you should use the food exchange diet system.

This exchange system will provide you with a diet that is nutritionally sound, flexible, easy to follow, and something you can live with the rest of your life.

Dieticians have developed this food exchange system to provide a nutritious, low-calorie diet while at the same time allowing for individual food preferences. The standard "Exchange Lists for Meal Planning" has been simplified for our recommended weight loss diet.[3]

Here's how the food exchange system works: All foods are classified into seven groups: (1) vegetables, (2) fruits, (3) breads, (4) meats, (5) milk, (6) beverages, fats, and sweets, and (7) unlimited foods. The fods within each group are approximately *the same in nutrients and calories.* (See Table 5-2 for the exchange lists.)

Each meal plan recommends a number of foods from each group, thus ensuring a balanced diet. Within each food group a person can interchange any foods according to personal preference, also ensuring a person maximum flexibility and choice. For example, let's assume a married couple are both on

[3]We thank the American Dietetic Association for permission to adapt their "Exchange List for Meal Planning" for our recommended weight loss diet. The exchange lists presented have been simplified and modified to make it easier to use as a weight loss diet. If you want the complete food exchange diet or want to reduce your fat intake as well as your calorie intake, then write the American Dietetic Association, 430 North Michigan Ave., Chicago, Illinois 60611, for a copy of their Exchange Lists for Meal Planning. If you have special dietary concerns, consult with your family physician.

a 1,200-calorie food plan that allows four bread and five meat exhanges a day. These two people can choose any food or combination of different foods from the bread exchange list as long as they don't total more than four bread exchanges. The wife might eat one slice of bread (one exchange), three quarters of a cup of unsweetened cereal (one exchange), two graham crackers (one exchange) and ½ cup mashed potato (one exchange), while the husband might choose a completely different combination of foods from the list that meets his food preferences.

Simply stated, foods within the same list can be substituted for each other, but foods from different exchange groups, in general, should not be substituted. A person needs to eat foods from each of the exchange lists to insure a balanced diet. For example, a 1,200-calorie meal plan calls for three fruit exchanges and four high-calorie fats, sweets, and beverage exchanges. You can eat any combination of foods from the fats, sweets, and beverages group worth four exchanges and any combination of foods from the fruit group worth three exchanges. However, you should not substitute three sweet exchanges for three fruit exchanges.

The food exchange lists have been developed for convenient, practical use, as well as for a balanced low-calorie diet. Therefore, the caloric values for the foods are only estimates and have often been rounded off. But for purposes of losing weight, they are sufficiently accurate.

TABLE 5–2
Food Exchange Lists

List 1: Vegetable Exchanges

One exchange of vegetables contains about 5 grams of carbohydrate, 2 grams of protein, and 25 calories.

A variety of vegetables, served either alone or in other foods such as casseroles, soups, or salads, contributes to sound health, vitality, and weight control. Dark green and deep yellow vegetables are among the leading sources of vitamin A. Many of the vegetables in the following group are notable sources of vitamin C: asparagus, broccoli, brussels sprouts, cabbage, cauliflower, collards, kale, dandelion, mustard and turnip greens, spinach, rutabagas, tomatoes and turnips. A number, including broccoli, brussels sprouts, beet greens, chard, and tomato juice, are particularly good sources of potassium. High folacin values are found in asparagus, beets, broccoli, brussels sprouts, cauliflower, collards, kale, and lettuce. Moderate amounts of vitamin B_6 are supplied by broccoli, brussels sprouts, cauliflower, collards, spinach, sauerkraut, tomatoes, and tomato juice. Fiber is present in all vegetables.

List 1A

The following raw vegetables may be used in any amount:

Celery	Lettuce
Chicory	Parsley
Chinese Cabbage	Radishes
Endive	Watercress
Escarole	

List 1B

This list shows the kinds of vegetables to use for one vegetable exchange. One exchange is ½ cup.

Asparagus	Greens (cont.):
Bean Sprouts	Mustard
Beets	Spinach
Broccoli	Turnip
Brussels Sprouts	Mushrooms
Cabbage	Okra
Carrots	Onions
Cauliflower	Rhubarb
Cucumbers	Rutabaga
Eggplant	Sauerkraut
Green Pepper	String Beans, green or yellow
Greens:	Summer Squash
Beet	Tomatoes
Chards	Tomato Juice
Collards	Turnips
Dandelion	Vegetable Juice Cocktail
Kale	Zucchini

Starchy vegetables are found in the Bread Exchange List.

List 2: Fruit Exchanges

One exchange of fruit contains about 10 grams of carbohydrates and 40 calories.

Everyone likes to buy fresh fruits in the height of their season. But you can also buy fresh fruits and can or freeze them for off-season use. For variety serve fruit as a salad or in combination with other foods for dessert.

Fruits are valuable for vitamins, minerals, and fiber. Vitamin C is abundant in citrus fruits and fruit juices and is found in raspberries, strawberries, mangoes, cantaloupes, honeydews, and papayas. The better sources of vitamin A among these fruits include fresh or dried apricots, mangoes, cantaloupes, nectarines, yellow peaches, and persimmons. Oranges, orange juice, and cantaloupe provide more folacin than most of the other fruits in this list. Many fruits are a valuable source of potassium, especially apricots, bananas, several of the berries, grapefruit, grapefruit juice, mangoes, cantaloupes, honeydews, nectarines, oranges, orange juice, and peaches.

Fruit may be used fresh, dried, canned, frozen, cooked, or raw, as long as *no* sugar is added.

This list shows the kinds and amounts of fruits to use for one fruit exchange.

Apple	1 small
Apple Juice	⅓ cup
Applesauce (unsweetened)	½ cup
Apricots, fresh	2 medium
Apricots, dried	4 halves
Banana	½ small
Berries	
Blackberries	½ cup
Blueberries	½ cup
Raspberries	½ cup
Strawberries	¾ cup
Cherries	10 large
Cider	⅓ cup
Dates	2
Figs, fresh	1
Figs, dried	1
Grapefruit	½
Grapes	12
Grape Juice	¼ cup
Mango	½ small

Melon	
Cantaloupe	¼ small
Honeydew	$^1/_8$ medium
Watermelon	1 cup
Nectarine	1 small
Orange	1 small
Orange Juice	½ cup
Papaya	¾ cup
Peach	1 medium
Pear	1 small
Persimmon, native	1 medium
Pineapple	½ cup
Pineapple Juice	⅓ cup
Plums	2 medium
Prunes	2 medium
Prune Juice	¼ cup
Raisins	2 tablespoons
Tangerine	1 medium

Cranberries may be used as desired if no sugar is added.

List 3: Bread Exchanges (Includes Bread, Cereal and Starchy Vegetables)

One exchange of bread contains about 15 grams of carbohydrates, 2 grams of protein, and 70 calories.

In this list, whole-grain and enriched breads and cereals, germ and bran products, and dried beans and peas are good sources of iron and among the better sources of thiamin. The whole-grain, bran, and germ products have more fiber than products made from refined flours. Dried beans and peas are also good sources of fiber. Wheat germ, bran, fried beans, potatoes, lima beans, parsnips, pumpkin, and winter squash are particularly good sources of potassium. The better sources of folacin in this listing include whole-wheat bread, wheat germ, dried beans, corn, lima beans, parsnips, green peas, pumpkin, and sweet potato.

Starchy vegetables are included in this list because they contain the same amount of carbohydrate and protein as one slice of bread.

This list shows the kinds and amounts of breads, cereals, starchy vegetables, and prepared foods to use for one bread exchange.

Bread	
White (including French and Italian)	1 slice
Whole-Wheat	1 slice
Rye or Pumpernickel	1 slice
Raisin	1 slice
Bagel, small	½

English Muffin, small   ½
Plain Roll, bread   1
Frankfurter Roll   ½
Hamburger Bun   ½
Dried Bread Crumbs   3 tbs.
Tortilla, 6″   1

Cereal
Bran Flakes   ½ cup
Other ready-to-eat unsweetened Cereal   ¾ cup
Puffed Cereal (unfrosted)   1 cup
Cereal (cooked)   ½ cup
Grits (cooked)   ½ cup
Rice or Barley (cooked)   ½ cup
Pasta (cooked)   ½ cup
 Spaghetti, Noodles, Macaroni
Popcorn (popped, no fat added)   3 cups
Cornmeal (dry)   2 tbs.
Flour   2½ tbs.
Wheat Germ   ¼ cup

Crackers
Arrowroot   3
Graham, 2½″ sq.   2
Matzoth, 4″ × 6″   ½
Oyster   20
Pretzels, 3⅛″ long × ⅛″ dia.   25
Rye Wafers, 2″ × 3½″   3
Saltines   6
Soda, 2½″ sq.   4

Dried Beans, Peas and Lentils
Beans, Peas, Lentils (dried and cooked)   ½ cup
Baked Beans, no pork (canned)   ¼ cup

Starchy Vegetables
Corn   ⅓ cup
Corn on Cob   1 small
Lima Beans   ½ cup
Parsnips   ⅔ cup
Peas, Green (canned or frozen)   ½ cup
Potato, White   1 small
Potato (mashed)   ½ cup
Pumpkin   ¾ cup
Winter Squash, Acorn or Butternut   ½ cup
Yam or Sweet Potato   ¼ cup

Prepared Foods

Biscuit 2 ″ dia.	1
(omit 1 Fat Exchange)	
Corn Bread, 2 ″ × 2 ″ × 1 ″	1
(omit 1 Fat Exchange)	
Corn Muffin, 2 ″ dia.	1
(omit 1 Fat Exchange)	
Crackers, round butter type	5
(omit 1 Fat Exchange)	
Muffin, plain small	1
(omit 1 Fat Exchange)	
Potatoes, French Fried, length 2 ″ to 3 ½ ″	8
(omit 1 Fat Exchange)	
Potato or Corn Chips	15
(omit 2 Fat Exchanges)	
Pancake, 5 ″ × ½ ″	1
(omit 1 Fat Exchange)	
Waffle, 5 ″ × ½ ″	1
(omit 1 Fat Exchange)	

List 4: Meat/Protein Exchanges

One exchange of lean meat contains about 7 grams of protein, 5 grams of fat, and 75 calories.

All of the foods in the meat exchange lists are good sources of protein, and many are also good sources of iron, zinc, vitamin B_{12} (present only in foods of animal origin) and other vitamins of the vitamin B-complex.

Cholesterol is of animal origin. Foods of plant origin have no cholesterol.

Oysters are outstanding for their high content of zinc. Crab, liver, trimmed lean meats, the dark muscle meat of turkey, dried beans and peas, and peanut butter all have much less zinc than oysters but are still good sources.

Dried beans, peas, and peanut butter are particularly good sources of magnesium and potassium.

You may use the meat, fish or other meat exchanges that are prepared for the family when no fat or flour has been added. If meat is fried, use the fat included in the Meal Plan. Meat juices with the fat removed may be used with your meat or vegetables for added flavor. Be certain to trim off all visible fat. The meat exchanges are divided into low-fat, medium-fat, and high-fat sublists. The low-fat list has both less calories and fats, and is considered healthier for you than the other two sublists of meats.

4A: Low-Fat Meats

This list shows the kinds and amounts of lean meat and other protein-rich foods to use for one low-fat meat exchange.

Beef:	Baby Beef (very lean), Chipped Beef, Chuck, Flank Steak, Tenderloin, Plate Ribs, Plate Skirt Steak, Round (bottom, top), all cuts Rump, Spare Ribs, Tripe	1 oz.
Lamb:	Leg, Rib, Sirloin, Loin (roast and chops), Shank, Shoulder	1 oz.
Pork:	Leg (Whole Rump, Center Shank), Ham, Smoked (center slices)	1 oz.
Veal:	Leg, Loin, Rib, Shank, Shoulder, Cutlets	1 oz.
Poultry:	Meat without skin of Chicken, Turkey, Cornish Hen, Guinea Hen, Pheasant	1 oz.
Fish:	Any fresh or frozen	1 oz.
	Canned Salmon, Tuna, Mackerel, Crab and Lobster	¼ cup
	Clams, Oysters, Scallops, Shrimp	5 or 1 oz.
	Sardines, drained	3
Cheeses containing less than 5% butterfat		1 oz.
Cottage Cheese, Dry and 2% butterfat		¼ cup
Dried Beans and Peas (omit 1 Bread Exchange)		½ cup

4B: Medium-Fat Meats

This list shows the kinds and amounts of medium-fat meat and other protein-rich foods to use for one medium-fat exchange.

Beef:	Ground (15% fat), Corned Beef (canned), Rib Eye, Round (ground commercial)	1 oz.
Pork:	Loin (all cuts Tenderloin), Shoulder Arm (picnic), Shoulder Blade, Boston Butt, Canadian Bacon, Boiled Ham	1 oz.
Liver, Heart, Kidney and Sweetbreads (these are high in cholesterol)		1 oz.
	Cottage Cheese, creamed	¼ cup
Cheese:	Mozzarella, Ricotta, Farmer's Cheese, Neufchatel, Parmesan	1 oz. 3 tbs.
Egg (high in cholesterol)		1
Peanut Butter (omit 2 additional Fat Exchanges)		2 tbs.

4C: High-Fat Meats

For each exchange of High-Fat Meat omit 1 Fat Exchange.

This list shows the kinds and amounts of high-fat meat and other protein-rich foods to use for one high-fat meat exchange.

Beef:	Brisket, Corned Beef (Brisket), Ground Beef (more than 20% *fat), Hamburger (commercial), Chuck (ground commercial), Roasts (Rib), Steaks (Club and Rib)*	1 oz.
Lamb:	Breast	1 oz.
Pork:	Spare Ribs, Loin (Back Ribs), Pork (ground), Country style Ham, Deviled Ham	1 oz.
Veal:	Breast	1 oz.
Poultry:	Capon, Duck (domestic), Goose	1oz.
Cheese:	Cheddar Types	1 oz.
Cold Cuts		$4\frac{1}{2}" \times$ $\frac{1}{8}"$ slice
Frankfurter		1 small

List 5: Milk Exchanges (include Non-Fat, Low-Fat and Whole Milk)

One exchange of milk contains about 12 grams of carbohydrate, 8 grams of protein, a trace of fat, and 80 calories.

Milk is a basic food for your Meal Plan for very good reasons. Besides the leading source of calcium, milk is a good source of phosphorus, protein, some of the B-complex vitamins, including folacin and vitamin B_{12}, and vitamins A and D. Magnesium is also found in milk.

Since it is a basic ingredient in many recipes you will not find it difficult to include milk in your Meal Plan. Milk can be used not only to drink but can be added to cereal, coffee, tea, and other foods.

This list shows the kinds and amounts of milk or milk products to use for milk exchange. They are divided into non-fat, low-fat, and whole milk.

Non-Fat Fortified Milk

Skim or non-fat milk	1 cup
Powdered (non-fat dry, before adding liquid)	⅓ cup
Canned, evaporated–skim milk	½ cup
Buttermilk made from skim milk	1 cup
Yogurt made from skim milk (plain, unflavored)	1 cup

Low-Fat Fortified Milk

2% fat fortified milk	¾ cup
Yogurt made from 2% fortified milk (plain, unflavored)	¾ cup

Whole Milk (Omit 2 Fat Exchanges)
    Whole milk   ½ cup
    Canned, evaporated whole milk   ¼ cup
    Buttermilk made from whole milk   ½ cup
    Yogurt made from whole milk (plain, unflavored)   ½ cup

*List 6: High Calorie Fats, Sweets, and Beverages Food Exchanges**

These foods contain about 45 calories.

The list shows the different amounts of foods and beverages to use for *one* food exchange. They are *high* in calories and low in nutrients, so be careful in their use.

For salads you may use mayonnaise or salad dressing as your fat exchange. For example, if you use 1 teaspoon of mayonnaise you would give up 1 teaspoon of butter. You may use your fat exchanges in preparing such foods as vegetables and meats. For example, if you use a teaspoon of fat to fry an egg, give up one exchange.

The sweets are very high in sugars and calories and very low or nonexistent in nutrients. They are sometimes called "empty" calories. The calories in sweets can add up very quickly, so measure your sweets carefully.

Alcoholic and nonalcoholic beverages have a suprisingly large number of calories. Enjoy your beverages, but drink in moderation as the calories and pounds can add up quickly.

For each exchange called for on your meal plan, choose any one item listed below in the amount given. Make sure you measure the exact amount you use because any more adds considerably to your caloric intake.

*Fats, sweets, and beverages have been combined into one food exchange list because they all contain large numbers of calories with few nutrients.

6A: Fats

This list shows the kinds and amounts of fat-containing foods to use for one fat exchange. To plan a diet low in saturated fat select only those exchanges that appear under polyunsaturated fats.

Polyunsaturated Fats		*Saturated Fats*	
Margarine, soft, tub or stick*	1 tsp	Margarine, regular stick	1 tsp.
Avocado (4″ in diameter)**	$^1/_8$	Butter	1 tsp.
Oil, Corn, Cottonseed, Safflower,		Bacon fat	1 tsp.
Soy, Sunflower	1 tsp	Bacon, crisp	1 strip
Oil, Olive**	1 tsp	Cream, light	2 tbs.
Oil, Peanut**	1 tsp	Cream, sour	2 tbs.
Olives**	5 small	Cream, heavy	1 tbs.
Almonds**	10 whole	Cream Cheese	1 tbs.
Pecans**	2 large whole	French dressing***	1 tbs.

Peanuts**		Italian dressing***	1 tbs.
Spanish	20 whole	Lard	1 tsp.
Virginia	10 whole	Mayonnaise***	1 tsp.
Walnuts	6 small	Salad dressing, mayonnaise	
Nuts, other**	6 small	type***	2 tsp.
		Salt pork	¾ cube

6B: Sweets

6C: Beverages

Cake, without icing	1 "	Beer	4 oz.
Cake, with icing	½ "	Carbonated beverages (e.g.,	
Candy	½ oz.	Coke)	4 oz.
Jam or Jelly	1 level tsp.	Liquor (gin, rum, whiskey)	
Pie 1 " piece of small pie		(⅓ jigger)	½ oz.
Sugar or Honey	1 level tbs.	Wine, light dry, 12%	2 oz.
Syrup	1 level tbs.	Wine, sweet, 20%	1 oz.

*Made with corn, cottonseed, safflower, soy or sunflower oil only.

**Fat content is primarily monounsaturated.

***If made with corn, cottonseed, safflower, soy or sunflower oil, can be used on fat-modified diet.

List 7: No-Calorie Unlimited Food Exchanges

At each meal, you may have any amount you wish from this list of foods, because these foods contain an insignificant number of calories. These foods do not need to be measured or recorded.

Unlimited

Bouillon (fat free)	Mustard (dry)
Clear broth	Pepper and other spices
Coffee (*without* milk or sugar)	Pickle (unsweetened)
Cranberries (unsweetened)	Rennet tablets
Gelatin (unsweetened)	Saccharin
Horseradish	Seasonings
Lemon	Tea (*without* milk or sugar)
Low-calorie soft drinks*	Vinegar

*Read the label—some are high in calories.

CALORIE MEAL PLANS

A meal plan specifies the number of total calories and number of food exchanges within each food group allowed per day. The higher the caloric value of the plan, the more exchanges are allowed. For example, a 1,000-calorie plan permits only three bread exchanges, but a 1,500-calorie plan allows five bread exchanges. Table 5–3 lists 1,000-, 1,200-, 1,500- and 1,800-calorie food plans. The calorie meal plans are set up to show the four common eating times—breakfast, lunch, dinner, and snacks—as well as the seven food lists. Each circle represents one food exchange, and each "AA" indicates that you can eat any amount of that specific food group. Thus each meal plan not only tells how many exchanges of each food group you can eat but also encourages you to eat three balanced meals a day. For example, look at the number of circles for each food group on the 1000-calorie meal plan. This plan allows any amount of A group vegetables and three vegetable exchanges of B group vegetables, three fruit exchanges, three bread exchanges, four meat exchanges, two milk exchanges, three high calorie fats, sugars, and beverage exchanges, and any amount of the unlimited exchanges. Looking across the different eating times, the 1,000 calorie meal plan encourages you to eat one fruit exchange for breakfast, lunch, and dinner; one bread exchange for breakfast, lunch, and dinner; one meat exchange for breakfast and lunch, and two meat exchanges for dinner; one milk exchange for breakfast and snack time, one high calorie fats, sweets, and beverage exchange for lunch, dinner, and snack; and any amount at any time of the last exchange.

Nutritionists do not recommend that people go below 1,000 calories a day as deficiencies in necessary nutrients can then occur. Nevertheless you can easily lose one to two pounds a week on a 1,000- or 1,200-calorie plan.

SELECTING YOUR CALORIE MEAL PLAN

An appropriate calorie meal plan depends primarily on how much weight you want to lose weekly. Assuming no increase in your physical activity (the subject of the next chapter), you have to reduce your calorie intake by 3,500 to lose one pound. Since generally a good weight loss is a steady one to two pounds a week, a reduction of 500 calories a day (3,500 calories a week) would give you a loss of approximately one pound a week; 1,000 calories a day (7,000 calories a week), would give you a loss of approximately two pounds a week. If your current food intake, for example, is about 2,500 calories a day, then you would have to reduce your intake by about 1,000 calories a day (to a total of 1,500 calories a day) to lose about two pounds per week.

TABLE 5-3
1,000-Calories Meal Plan

	Breakfast	*Lunch*	*Dinner*	*Snack*
1. Vegetable Exchanges A any amount(AA) B 25 calories	AA	AA O	AA O O	AA
2. Fruit Exchanges 40 calories	O	O	O	
3. Bread Exchanges 70 calories	O	O	O	
4. Meat Exchanges 75 calories	O	O	O	
5. Milk Exchanges 80 calories	O			O
6. High Calorie Fats, Sweets & Beverages Exchanges 45 calories		O	O	O
7. No Calorie Unlimited Exchanges 0 calories Any amount (AA)	AA	AA	AA	AA

1,200-Calorie Meal Plan

	Breakfast	*Lunch*	*Dinner*	*Snack*
1. Vegetable Exchanges A any amount (AA) B 25 calories	AA	AA O	AA O O	AA
2. Fruit Exchanges 40 calories	O	O	O	

TABLE 5-3 *(cont.)*

	Breakfast	Lunch	Dinner	Snack
3. Bread Exchanges 　70 calories	○	○	○○	
4. Meat Exchanges 　75 calories	○	○	○○○	
5. Milk Exchanges 　80 calories	○			○
6. High Calorie Fats, 　Sweets, & Beverages 　Exchanges 　45 calories	○	○	○	○
7. No Calorie Unlimited 　Exchanges 　0 calories 　Any amount (AA)	AA	AA	AA	AA

1,500-Calorie Meal Plan

	Breakfast	Lunch	Dinner	Snack
1. Vegetable Exchanges 　A　any amount (AA) 　B　25 calories	AA	AA ○	AA ○○	AA
2. Fruit Exchanges 　40 calories	○	○○	○	
3. Bread Exchanges 　70 calories	○	○	○○	○
4. Meat Exchanges 　75 calories	○	○○○	○○○	
5. Milk Exchanges 　80 calories	○			○
6. High Calorie Fats, 　Sweets, & Beverages 　Exchanges 　45 calories	○	○	○○	○
7. No Calorie Unlimited 　Exchanges 　0 calories 　Any amount (AA)	AA	AA	AA	AA

TABLE 5-3 *(cont.)*

1,800-Calorie Meal Plan

	Breakfast	Lunch	Dinner	Snack

1. Vegetable Exchanges
   A Any amount (AA)
   B 25 calories
	AA	AA
		O
		O
			AA
			O
			O
			O
				AA

2. Fruit Exchanges 40 calories	O	O O	O O	
3. Bread Exchanges 70 calories	O	O O	O O	O
4. Meat Exchanges 85 calories	O	O O O	O O O	
5. Milk Exchanges 80 calories	O			O

6. High Calorie Fats,
   Sweets, & Beverages
   Exchanges
   45 calories
	O
	O
		O
		O
			O
			O
				O

7. No Calorie Unlimited
   Exchanges
   0 calories
   Any amount (AA)
	AA	AA	AA	AA

To determine your calorie meal plan, check your estimated daily calorie intake as recorded in your eating diary described in Chapter 3. Then subtract 500 or 1,000 calories from your estimated daily calorie intake to obtain your estimated meal plan. For example, Susan estimated her daily calorie intake at 2,000 calories and wanted to lose about one pound a week. She subtracted 500 calories from her daily caloric intake of 2,000 calories, leaving 1,500 calories for her estimated calorie meal plan.

Susan's Estimated Daily Calorie Intake	2000 calories
Subtract 500 calories a day (for 1 pound a week)	500 calories
or	
1000 calories a day (for 2 pounds a week)	____
Susan's estimated calorie meal plan =	1500 calories

Fill in the following blanks to obtain your food plan:

Your estimated daily calorie intake	_____	calories
Subtract 500 calories a day (for 1 pound a week)	_____	calories
1,000 calories a day (for 2 pounds a week)	_____	calories
Your estimated calorie meal plan	_____	calories

Try this meal plan for two to three weeks and see how much weight you lose. You may need to decrease or increase the caloric value to meet your weight loss goals and hunger needs. We strongly recommend this experimental "try-and-see" approach to see what works best for you. Usually a 1,200- or 1,500-calorie diet provides an optimal weight loss. If you did *not* estimate your daily caloric intake, or if you think your estimate is inaccurate, then start with a 1,200-calorie meal plan and adjust it as needed after trying it for several weeks.

AN EXAMPLE OF A FOOD EXCHANGE DIET

You must become familiar with the different food groups and their approximate food values. Initially you must measure all the food you eat and continue to do so until you become very accurate in estimating the quantity. If you don't already have measuring spoons and cups, buy them and use them. When you shop for meat, note the weights on the packages. You can even buy a little postage or food scale to weigh your food. Since there is an understandable tendency to *under*estimate quantity and caloric value, whenever in doubt, be safe and round off to the higher number!

For the first week, record all the foods you eat and practice converting them to the food exchange system. To illustrate more clearly how to do this, we have provided a list of the food eaten on Tuesday by Bobby, who is on a 1,500-calorie diet (Table 5-4). Based on the food lists, place an "X" in the appropriate circle that represents the food eaten by Bobby, also write the name of the food beneath the "X". Try to do this *without* looking at the following table, to get some practice.

TABLE 5-4
Food Eaten by Bobby on Tuesday

Breakfast	*Dinner*
½ small grapefruit	1 baked potato
¾ cup unsweetened cereal	1 cup spinach
1 cup skim milk	1 cup skim milk
Tea, with 1 tablespoon sugar	3 oz. lean steak
	1 teaspoon margarine
Lunch	1 tablespoon sugar
1 slice whole wheat bread	1 cup squash
¼ cup cottage cheese	coffee
¼ medium-sized cantaloupe	salt, pepper, seasonings
½ cup pineapple	
3 celery sticks	*Snack*
2 oz. lean hamburger	½ cup skim milk
1 cup clear broth	3 vanilla wafers
	6 peanuts

After you have filled in the 1,500-calorie Meal Plan, look at Bobby's 1,500-calorie meal diary for the day (Table 5-5). Bobby ate for breakfast one-half of a grapefruit, three-fourths of a cup of cereal, one cup skim milk, and tea with one tablespoon of sugar. The food exchange lists indicate that one-half of a grapefruit equals one fruit exchange, so Bobby placed a "X" in the circle under Fruit Exchanges/Breakfast; three-fourths of a cup of cereal equals one bread exchange, so Bobby placed an "X" in the circle under Bread Exchange/Breakfast; one cup of skim milk equals one milk exchange so Bobby placed an "X" in the circle under Milk Exchange/Breakfast; one tablespoon of sugar equals one sweet exchange so Bobby placed an "X" in the circle under High Calorie Fats, Sweets, and Beverages Ex-

TABLE 5-5
Bobby's 1,500-Calorie Meal Diary

	Total Calories	Breakfast	Lunch	Dinner	Snack
1. Vegetable Exchanges		AA	AA	AA (spinach)	AA
A Any amount				⊗(squash, 1cup)	
B 25 calories ×2 =	50		○(celery)		
2. Fruit Exchanges		⊗(grapefruit ½)	⊗(cantaloupe ½) ⊗(pineapple ½ c.) ○		
40 calories ×3 =	120				
3. Bread Exchanges		⊗(cereal, ¾ cup)	⊗(bread, 1 slice)	○(potato, 1 med)(wafers, 3)	
70 calories ×4 =	280				
4. Meat Exchanges		○	⊗(cottage cheese ¼c.)(hamburger, 2 oz.)	⊗(steak, 3 oz.)	
75 calories ×6 =	450				
5. Milk Exchanges		⊗(1 cup skim milk)		⊗(skim milk, 1 cup)(skim milk 1c)	
80 calories ×3 =	240				
6. High Calorie Fats, Sweets, & Beverages Exchanges		⊗(sugar, 1 tbs.) ○		⊗(sugar, 1 tbs.)(margarine,) ⊗(peanuts, 6)(wafers, 1tb)	
45 calories ×4 =	180				
7. No Calorie Unlimited Exchanges		AA (tea)	AA (water)	AA (coffee)(seasonings)	AA
0 calories Any amount (AA)					
Total Exchanges Calories	1,320				
Additional Calories	0				
Total Calories	1,320				

108

changes/Breakfast. Bobby also placed "X"s in the circles indicating the food he ate for lunch, dinner and his snack as well.

To determine his total caloric consumption for the day, Bobby multiplied the number of calories for a food group exchange by the number of exchanges eaten in that group. For example, one vegetables exchange equals 25 calories multiplied by 2 exchanges equals 50 calories. He then added together the total calories consumed in each food group to obtain his total calorie consumption for the day, which was 1,320 calories.

Bobby ate balanced, varied meals that met his individual preferences, prevented feelings of hunger, and kept his caloric intake to 1,320 calories (this diet plan calls for eating 1,500 *or* less). Thus, Bobby was successful that day in controlling his caloric intake and accordingly felt good and rewarded himself.

In planning your diet, try to eat three meals a day and have foods from each food exchange group. These, however, are general guidelines, *not rigid rules.* For example, not having a meat for breakfast is acceptable; simply eat a meat exchange at another meal. Some limited shifting of foods from one exchange to another exchange is also fine, if they are about equal in calories. For example, Bobby selected one additional milk exchange and one less meat exchange than called for. One should *not* however, substitute fats, sweets and beverages for fruits and vegetables.

Though eating is something we must do to survive, fortunately it can also be an enjoyable and even tasty experience. But eating can—and should be—even more enjoyable by learning how to eat well without gaining weight. The general guideline is *to eat in moderation but to enjoy what you eat.* To this end we have included a seven-day menu plan in Appendix C to show you some of the tasty, low-calorie, and filling meals you can eat. Try these recipes and add your own. For additional tips on low-calorie cooking, try some of the cook books listed in the references.

SELF-OBSERVING YOUR FOOD
EXCHANGE DIET

In Chapter 2 we emphasized the importance of increased awareness and self-observing to understand and control your behavior. To keep you aware of your intake, observing and writing down what you eat is very helpful. We have therefore developed a convenient weekly diet monitoring system, in the form of food lists, which are summarized each on one page in Appendix D. Cut that page out along the dotted lines and carry it with you or tape it to the refrigerator door.

In Appendix E, there is a Weekly Calorie Intake Diary of each food calorie plan. Again, cut out the food calorie plan you have selected and make ten photocopies of that page. You now have a convenient way to record your daily intake for ten weeks. When you need additional record sheets, simply keep one blank copy and make more copies from it. Carry the weekly calorie intake sheets with you or tape them on the refrigerator door or another convenient location. After each meal, check off the food exchanges you have consumed and then total the calories consumed at the end of the day. Remember: record the calories as soon as possible—we all have ways of "forgetting" things quickly.

If some combinations of foods are difficult to break down into the designated food exchange groups, then simply look up the caloric value in a calorie book and insert the number of calories under the selection labelled, "Additional Calories."[4] Include these in the total calories consumed during the day.

At the end of the week you will have a record of your daily

---

[4]Two books on counting calories are: Kraus, *Calories and Carbohydrates* (1973) and United States Department of Agriculture, *Calories and Weight* (1968).

fluctuations. Some people prefer to continue recording everything they eat, which is fine. The important point is to keep aware of what you eat as a way to permanently change your eating habits.

SUMMARY

At the beginning of this chapter, we talked about the need for changes in your eating and activity habits in ways that you can live with the rest of your life. To better understand the food you eat, we presented basic facts about proteins, carbohydrates, fats, vitamins, and minerals. If you selected a structured food exchange diet of seven, well-balanced food groups, you can tailor a meal plan of 1,000, 1,200, 1,500, or 1,800 calories a day, depending on your present intake and weight loss goal.

The program sounds easier than it actually is. The permanent changes you are looking for are not easy and will not come quickly. You will need time, work, and discipline.

To keep your spirits up and your weight down, however, physical exercise always helps. Proper diet and reasonable activity give you two forces working on the energy balance in your body: you are taking in fewer calories to start with, and burning off a few more to boot.

Let's look into the subject of physical activities in the next chapter.

6

Using Up Calories and Physical Activity

Many weight problems begin with a lack of proper exercise. Becoming more physically active helps to take pounds off. So in this chapter, we are going to talk about physical activity. As we do, take a close look at your own exercise habits: How much exercise do you get each day? If necessary we will help you develop a plan to increase your exercise level; we will also give you some practical suggestions to implement that plan and keep it going.

BENEFITS OF PHYSICAL ACTIVITY

EXERCISE BURNS CALORIES

If your eating patterns remain unchanged, you can still gain weight by a reduction in energy outflow. This reduction may result from a lowering of basal metabolism, which occurs gradually with age, or from a decline in day-to-day activity.

Growing older is something beyond control: It happens naturally, and there is little you can do about it. Physical activity, however, is something you can control. By increasing your daily activity level you automatically burn off more calories. As you know, one pound of fat equals approximately 3,500 calories, thus for every 3,500 calories you burn, you come one pound closer to your weight loss goal. Given a moderate diet, the more calories used in exercise, the more pounds you lose and the easier it is to maintain your weight as well.

Most people are unaware of the number of calories they expend by performing daily activities. You can test your own knowledge by estimating how many calories the average person uses while doing each of the following activities for approximately ten minutes. *After* you have completed the table below, check the accuracy of your answers at the bottom of the page.[1]

Activity for 10 minutes	*Estimated caloric expenditure*
1. Sleeping	
2. Watching TV	
3. Light gardening	
4. Taking a leisurely bike ride	
5. Walking outdoors	
6. Playing tennis	

Have you checked your answers? If you are like most people, your estimates were probably too high. Burning off excessive weight takes more time and effort then you thought.

The exact number of calories expended per unit of exercise varies among people depending upon such factors as size and sex. For example, Table 6–1 provides an estimate of the caloric expenditure for various activities performed by medium-sized men and women. A careful look at the table will give you a

---

[1] *Answers:* (Approximate number of calories used per ten minutes of the above activities.) Sleeping = 12; Watching TV = 14; Light gardening = 40; Bike riding = 70; Walking outdoors = 61; Playing tennis = 70.

good idea of the amount of time it takes to burn off 3,500 calories, or to lose one pound.

Lest you become discouraged, remember that the effects of exercise are *cumulative* and that the estimates are based on *only one minute of activity.* So if, for example, you got into the habit of taking a brisk thirty-minute walk each day, in a year you would lose almost eighteen pounds from this activity alone. Figure at 4 m.p.h., you expend 5.8 calories per minute. Over 30 minutes, you expend 174 calories (30 × 5.8). In 365 days, the calorie count accumulates to 63,410 calories. Divide that total by 3,500, and you find you've burned off about 18 pounds (63,410 ÷ 3,500 = 18.1 pounds).

To better understand the effects of exercise, it is helpful to know the *exercise equivalents* of various foods. Exercise equivalents show the amount of time needed in an activity to use up the food you have eaten. Stated differently, you might ask yourself what you will need to do in the way of exercise to compensate for "fat" foods and snacks. You will find the answers in Table 6-2.

EXERCISE REDUCES YOUR APPETITE

A misconception shared by many people is that when exercise increases, so does appetite. Many believe that we *must* compensate for physical activity by becoming hungrier and eating more. This belief is untrue. In fact, research studies indicate just the opposite: Hunger actually *decreases* with moderate activity. You may even lose your appetite temporarily if you exercise to the point of exhaustion.

Jean Mayer, a distinguished nutritionist at Harvard University, has conducted several studies on the role of activity in hunger and obesity with both animals and humans as subjects. Mayer found that animals (in this case, laboratory rats) with lowered activity levels actually ate more than those with normal activity levels. Under conditions of normal activity the

TABLE 6-1
Calories Used in Physical Activities*

	Calories per min.		Calories per min.
I. Resting, Standing and Walking			
Kneeling	1.4	Standing, light activity	2.8
Resting in bed	1.2	Walking, 2 mph	3.2
Sitting	1.4	Walking, 3 mph	4.4
Sitting, watching TV	1.4	Walking, 4 mph	5.8
Sitting, eating	1.6	Walking, downstairs	7.6
Sitting, playing cards	1.7	Walking, upstairs	20.0
Standing	1.6	Washing and dressing	2.6
II. Working Around the Home			
Beds, making	5.3	Machine sewing	1.5
Dusting	2.5	Peeling vegetables	2.9
Floors, mopping	5.3	Shaking carpets	6.4
Floors, sweeping	1.7	Stirring, mixing foods	3.0
Ironing clothes	4.2	Washing clothes	2.9
Laundry	4.0	Window cleaning	3.5
III. Do It Yourself			
Carrying tools	3.6	Pushing wheelbarrow	5.2
Chopping wood	4.9	Sawing wood	6.9
Drilling	7.0	Shoveling	7.9
Gardening, digging	8.6	Stacking wood	6.1
Planing wood	8.6		
IV. Sports			
Badminton	2.8	Horseback riding	3.0
Basketball	8.6	Jogging	10.0
Bowling	18.1	Ping-Pong	4.9
Canoeing, moderate	4.0	Playing pool	3.0
Cycling	8.0	Rowing	8.0
Dancing	4.0	Sailing	2.6
Football	10.1	Skiing, cross country	11.0
Golfing	5.5	Sprinting	23.3
Handball, squash	10.2	Swimming	12.1
Hiking, flat	5.0	Tennis	7.0
Hiking, mountain	10.0		
V. Occupations			
Assembly work	2.3	Mixing, Cement	6.3
Automobile repair	4.2	Painting	3.5
Carpentry	3.8	Standing, light activity	2.6
Classwork, studying	1.1	Typing, electric	1.5
Farming	3.8		

*Adapted from J. Mayer, *31 Days to a Slimmer You* © 1975 The News, Inc., World rights reserved. See Durnin and Passmore (1967) for more information about energy expenditure in physical activities.

TABLE 6-2

Energy Equivalents of Food Calories Expressed in Minutes of Activity*

Food	Calories	Walking[1]	Riding bicycle[2]	Swimming[3]	Running[4]	Reclining[5]
Apple, large	101	19	12	9	5	78
Bacon, 2 strips	96	18	12	9	5	74
Banana, small	88	17	11	8	4	68
Beans, green, 1 c.	27	5	3	2	1	21
Beer, 1 glass	111	22	14	10	6	88
Bread and butter	78	15	10	7	4	60
Cake, 2-layer, 1/12	356	68	43	32	18	274
Carbonated beverage, 1 glass	106	20	13	9	5	82
Carrot, raw	42	8	5	4	2	32
Cereal, dry, ½ c. with milk, sugar	200	38	24	18	10	154
Cheese, cottage 1 tbsp.	27	5	3	2	1	21
Cheese, Cheddar, 1 oz.	111	21	14	10	6	85
Chicken, fried, ½ breast	232	45	23	21	12	173
Chicken, TV Dinner	542	104	66	48	28	417
Cookie, plain	15	3	2	1	1	12
Cookie, chocolate chip	51	10	6	5	3	39
Doughnut	151	29	18	13	8	116
Egg, fried	110	21	13	10	3	85
Egg, boiled	77	15	9	7	3	45
French dressing, 1 tbsp.	59	11	7	5	3	45
Halibut steak, ¼ lb.	205	39	25	10	11	158
Ham, 2 slices	167	32	20	15	9	128
Ice cream, 1/6 qt.	193	37	24	17	10	148

Table 6–2 (*cont.*)

Food	Calories	*Minutes of Activity*				
		Walk-ing[1]	Riding bicycle[2]	Swim-ming[3]	Run-ning[4]	Re-clining[5]
Ice cream soda	255	49	31	23	13	196
Ice milk, $^1/_6$ qt.	144	28	18	13	7	111
Gelatin, with cream	117	23	14	10	6	90
Malted milk shake	502	97	61	45	25	386
Mayonnaise, 1 tbsp.	92	18	11	8	5	71
Milk, 1 glass	166	32	20	15	9	128
Milk, skim, 1 glass	81	16	10	7	4	62
Milk shake	421	81	51	38	22	324
Orange, medium	68	13	8	6	4	32
Orange juice, 1 glass	120	23	15	11	6	92
Pancake with syrup	124	24	13	11	6	95
Peach, medium	46	9	6	4	2	35
Peas, green, ½ c.	56	11	7	5	3	43
Pie, apple, $^1/_6$	377	73	46	34	19	290
Pie, raisin, $^1/_6$	437	84	53	39	23	316
Pizza, cheese, $^1/_8$	180	35	22	16	9	188
Pork chop, loin	314	60	38	28	16	242
Potato chips, 1 serving	108	21	13	10	6	83
Sandwiches:						
Club	590	113	72	53	30	454
Hamburger	350	67	43	31	18	260
Roast beef with gravy	430	83	52	38	22	331
Tuna fish salad	278	53	34	25	14	214
Sherbet, $^1/_6$ qt.	177	34	22	16	9	136
Shrimp, French fried	180	35	22	16	9	138
Spaghetti, 1 serving	396	76	48	35	20	306
Steak, T-bone	235	45	29	21	12	181
Strawberry shortcake	400	77	49	36	21	308

[1]Energy cost of walking for 50-lb. individual = 5.2 calories per minute at 35 m.p.h.
[2]Energy cost of riding bicycle = 8.3 calories per minute.
[3]Energy cost of swimming = 11.2 calories per minute.
[4]Energy cost of running = 19.4 calories per minute.
[5]Energy cost of reclining = 1.3 calories per minute.

*From: Konishi, F. Food energy equivalents of various activities. *Journal American Dietetic Association,* 1965, *46,* 186. Used with permission.

animals voluntarily adjusted their caloric intake to meet energy requirements; they also maintained their weight. However, when the animals were required to be sedentary (that is, their activity level was lowered for purposes of the experiment), they did not make corresponding adjustments in caloric intake and their weight *increased*.

Similar findings have been obtained with people. For example, in one study the eating and activity habits of three hundred white and blue collar workers were examined[2] (see Figure 6–1 for a summary of the results). As you can see from the figure, the lowest food intake was by workers who engaged in light but regular work. Sedentary workers ate *more* than those engaged in light, medium, or heavy work and were also the *heaviest* of all of the workers studied. These results suggest that, contrary to popular belief, *moderate* amounts of regular exercise can have the beneficial effect of *helping you eat less*.

EXERCISE IMPROVES
THE SHAPE YOU'RE IN

Regular exercise not only helps you lose weight, but it also strengthens unused muscles, builds better muscle tone, coordination, strength, shape, and confidence in your body. Our bodies are made to be exercised, and they look and feel better when they are.

EXERCISE
IMPROVES YOUR HEALTH

Regular exercise promotes digestion, improves circulation, lowers fat and cholesterol levels in the blood, and improves the functioning of the heart.[3] Since problems in these areas are

[2]See Mayer (1968) for the details.

[3]Mayer, J. *Overweight* (Englewood Cliffs, N.J.: Prentice Hall, 1968).

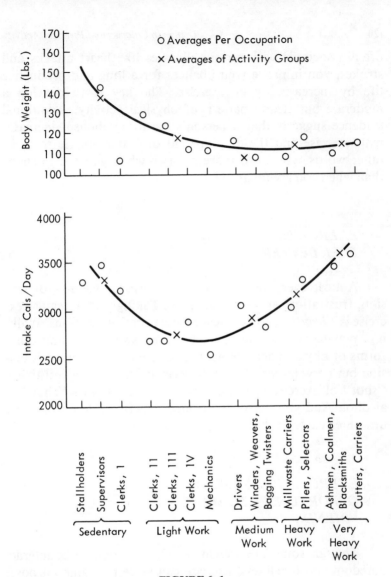

FIGURE 6–1.

Body weight and caloric intake as a function of physical activity in man. In a study by Mayer (1968 p. 74) the voluntary food intake of 300 workers was investigated. Note that the lowest voluntary food intake is seen in workers who engage in light regular activity. Sedentary workers eat more and are much fatter. Workers performing heavy work eat more but their weight is still light. Used with permission, Prentice-Hall, Inc.

often associated with serious illnesses like heart attacks and strokes, you improve your chances for a long and productive life by increasing your exercise. The key is to develop a moderate but steady pattern of physical activity. Additional evidence suggests that a person's basal metabolism increases with exercise and the development of better muscle tone. In other words, you burn more calories when you are in shape than when you are fat and flabby.

EXERCISE MAKES YOU
FEEL BETTER

Almost everyone experiences occasional feelings of tension, frustration, anxiety, and anger. Taking part in regular exercise is a *healthy* way to release these negative emotions. Walking, playing tennis, bicycling, bowling, swimming, and other forms of physical activity help to reduce not only nervous tension but nervous eating as well. Recent findings suggest that a "shot" of exercise will relax you even more than a "shot" of alcohol. And you derive this added benefit while burning off unwanted calories.

EXERCISE PROVIDES AN
OPPORTUNITY TO MAKE
FRIENDS

Though some overweight people use food to counteract boredom and loneliness, exercise can serve the same purpose. For example, participating in sports can provide entertainment and the opportunity to meet people, to socialize, and to form friendships. In the process you will be losing weight, not putting it on.

EXERCISE HELPS SOLVE THE
ENERGY CRISIS

Today two energy crises exist—the *personal* and the *societal* crises. The personal energy crisis is the result of individuals' not using *enough* of the fat energy stored in their bodies. The societal crisis is the result of individuals using *too much* energy drawn from our dwindling natural resources.

In the societal energy crunch, a large source of energy remains untapped in society—the adipose tissue of millions of people. Approximately 70 million Americans are overweight: If we assume they are, on the average, ten pounds overweight (a conservative estimate), they therefore carry 700 million pounds of fat. If 3,500 calories constitute a pound, then overweight Americans carry over 2,450 billion calories of energy in their fat cells.

How can we use this energy source and save our precious gasoline? The state of Oregon is already indirectly and partially solving this problem by allocating one percent of gasoline taxes for building safe and convenient bike paths. By increasing your bicycling and walking, both for recreation *and* for transportation, you burn off fat, reduce weight, release tension, decrease appetite, improve cardiovascular conditioning, decrease air pollution, and reduce gasoline consumption.

Although many benefits are to be gained, we realize exercising is not an easy habit to establish. You must change your beliefs and attitudes about exercise. Exercise does not have to mean a lot of hard and time-consuming work; even giving up a few electric gadgets you may have become accustomed to is a start. Do you really need that electric toothbrush? But the payoff more than exceeds the cost—in terms of faster weight loss, better health, improved appearance, more vitality, and zest for living. When you think about it, that amounts to quite a bargain.

WHAT ARE YOUR CURRENT
PHYSICAL ACTIVITY HABITS?

If the preceding discussion has encouraged you to begin a regular exercise program, good! That was our intent. More important, you will be doing yourself a favor. But a pledge to change is easier said than done. So where do you go from here?

Take a good look at your *present* level of activity. Knowing what you *want to do* is always easier if you know where to start. So for a starter, look at the physical activity questionnaire you completed in Chapter 3 (Table 3-5); it should give you a general estimate of your *present* activity level.

For a more precise idea of your present activity level, use the physical activity record in Appendix F. For the next week or two jot down all your physical activities (exclude resting, sleeping, lying down, and sitting), as well as the amount of time you spend doing them. After completing this log, you can calculate the number of calories you've burned by locating the various activities in the caloric expenditure chart (Table 6-1). Adding the numbers up each day will give you a reasonable estimate of the number of calories you expend daily in physical activity.

Once you know how many calories you presently burn, the next question is how many more do you want to burn to lose weight? Some people think they have to do strenuous exercises every day before they can benefit from an exercise program. Though they vow to follow a demanding Spartan regimen, within a week or two they understandably revert to a sedentary life style. Too much too soon is the problem.

To avoid this happening to you, answer these few questions about your own life style and interests. Your answers to the questions can guide you in selecting an exercise program that is *convenient, enjoyable,* and *likely to endure.*

1. Have you talked with your family doctor to discover if there are any medical reasons to avoid or to take up certain types of exercise? Yes_____ No_____. We strongly recommend that you receive your physician's approval before starting a new exercise program.

2. Do you have the time to exercise? Yes_____ No_____. If yes, how much time (in minutes) do you have daily? Can you make time to exercise?

3. Do you have a gym, park, or recreation facilities nearby your home or work? Yes_____ No_____.

4. Do you like to exercise alone? Yes_____ No_____.

5. Do you like to exercise with a friend or group? Yes_____ No_____.

6. If your answer to Question 5 was yes, could you ask one of your friends to begin exercising with you? Yes_____ No_____.

7. What types of physical activity have you enjoyed doing in the past?_____

8. Is there any reason why you can't take them up again? Yes_____ No_____.

9. Have you considered any new forms of activity that you think you might enjoy doing? Yes_____ No_____.

SOME POSSIBLE PHYSICAL ACTIVITIES FOR YOU

When you think about it, the activities people can do are almost unlimited. Some of them are hard, others easy. Some take special equipment, while others do not. Some require other people, but others can be done alone. Some take considerable practice to be good, but others can be done by almost anyone with little practice. All of them, however, require energy to perform. Doing them burns calories.

Below we suggest various exercises and activities that can be done easily at home, at work, while traveling, or as a recreational outlet. Except for recreation, most of them are not strenuous, nor do they burn off a lot of calories each time they are performed. But, remember, the good effects of exercise are cumulative: When they are done regularly, the number of calories you expend adds up quickly.

AT HOME

Instead of using electrical energy, get in the habit of using your body energy to brush your teeth, mix food, open cans, cut food, mow the lawn, trim the hedge, and so forth. By using your own energy, you not only burn off more calories, but save money and energy too. With today's high costs, especially for energy, that's not a bad deal.

Other household activities include: (1) walking up or down the stairs whenever things need to be done, rather than putting them off until later; (2) cleaning, washing, sweeping around the house; and (3) maintaining your own vegetable or flower garden. All these require extra energy to perform.

Another pleasant way to aid your diet is through increased sexual activity. Obviously, of the many dimensions of sex, the physical activity itself is usually enjoyable enough so that most people don't require special reminders to engage in it. Depending on the duration and amount of movement during "sexercises," your caloric expenditure can range from 50 to 250 calories per sexual encounter.

AT WORK

If you work in a building with more than one floor, get in the habit of using the stairs instead of the elevator. Even if you work in a high-rise building, you can exit the elevator a couple of floors below your office and walk the rest of the way. With time, you can climb more and more stairs. Walking or running upstairs and up hills are among the most efficient ways to use calories *and* strengthen the entire cardiovascular system.

Have you ever considered taking a mid-morning and mid-afternoon activity break? Instead of sitting over coffee and doughnuts, try walking around the block with a friend, doing a few stretching exercises (see the end of this chapter), even shooting some baskets at the company gym. Just standing up occasionally burns off more calories than sitting continuously. Another office exercise is to grab the seat of your chair and lift your body by pressing down with your hands and arms. Doing this a few times gets your circulation going and strengthens your arm and shoulder muscles.

TRANSPORTATION

All of us travel to perform work, to go shopping, to engage in recreational activities, and so forth. While the automobile is a real convenience in meeting transportation needs, cars are used excessively. Many activities close to home can be just as easily reached by walking or bicycling—a discovery you may have made during the dramatic gasoline shortage of 1974. Perhaps you should consider walking or biking the next time you reach for the car keys to travel to a nearby place. Over-reliance on the family car is a difficult habit to break, but by walking or bicycling you conserve gas, save money, help provide a cleaner environment, and reduce tension and weight as well.

RECREATION

Spectator sports are a popular American pastime, but we burn very few calories by participating in athletics vicariously. In fact, between the vending man at the stadium and the refrigerator near the TV, *gaining weight* is easy while watching others perform. On the other hand, countless other activities are easily learned and fun to do, such as swimming, tennis, hik-

ing, golf, volleyball, badminton, bowling, basketball, canoe-
ing, boating, baseball, dancing, and jogging. Many of them can
be performed alone without much advance preparation, while
others can be done with friends and teammates for social enjoyment. In all cases they are better for you than inactivity or arm-
chair athletics.

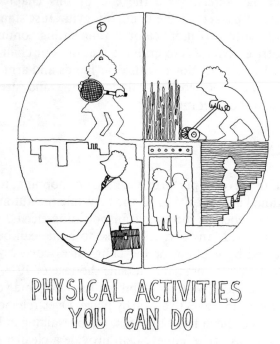

PHYSICAL ACTIVITIES
YOU CAN DO

Courtesy of Dannon Milk Products. Used by permission.

PLANNING YOUR OWN
EXERCISE PROGRAM

Now that you have determined your present activity level
and some possible activities available to you, let's plan an exercise program. To get you started, consider the results of one
person's planning in Table 6–3; it seems to provide a sound and

TABLE 6-3
Laura's Planned Physical Activities: An Example

Activity	Calories Expended per minute	× Minutes per Week Doing Activity	= Total Calories Used per Activity
1. Bicycling	8	30 minutes	240
2. Walking up and down stairs	13.8	(5 min. per day x 7 =) 35 minutes	483
3. Walking moderately outdoors	6.1	(15 min. per day x 7=)105 minutes	640.5
4. Tennis	7.0	60 minutes	420
5. Gardening	8.6	60 minutes	516
6. Making Love	5.3	30 minutes (Actual time spent making love, not lying in bed afterward.)	159
Total			2458.5

sensible approach. Notice Laura starts off modestly; the amount of exercise can always be *increased gradually* as she gets into better shape. Further, the activities she selected are compatible with her daily activities. She didn't need a large chunk of time each day because she chose several light activities that could be performed in a variety of settings—at home (gardening), at work (using the stairs), in transport (walking and cycling), as well as during leisure time (playing tennis). While these activities may not sound like much, they represent an improvement over Laura's previous sedentary life patterns. They also amount to over 2,400 calories per week in expended energy, or converted to weight loss, approximately .7 pounds a week or about *thirty-six pounds in a year's time.* There are no fads or frills involved, just a modest proposal put into regular practice. Developing a similar program can work equally well for you.

Start by selecting activities that you *can* do but that you don't do presently. Select activities that you enjoy *and* that use energy; the more calories they require the better. Estimate how long, in minutes, you plan to do each one during the week. Virtually any activity you aren't doing now will increase your total energy expenditure. Thus, if the activity is practical and to your liking, include it on your list. Write each of these activities in Table 6–4, "Your Planned Physical Activities."

Then take another look at Table 6–1 on calories used in various activities and get the number of calories expended per minute for each of your activities. Multiply the number of minutes per week for each of your listed activities by the number of calories per minute. By adding the calories for each activity, you will obtain an estimated number of calories burned off each week from your program. When you see what you have to gain (and it won't be more pounds!) by going ahead with your plan, you may feel encouraged to try it.

See how your ideas work for a week or more before going on with the reading.

TABLE 6-4

Your Planned Physical Activities

Activity	Calories Expended Per Minute	× Minutes Per Week	= Total Calories Expended Per Activity
1.			
2.			
3.			
4.			
5.			
6.			
7.			

Total Calories
Expended per Week = _____

EXERCISE UPDATE
AND A PHYSICAL ACTIVITY DIARY

How has your exercise program been going? Some of your activities were probably performed flawlessly, just as you had hoped. For this we offer our congratulations. You too should feel good about that and remember to reward yourself accordingly. Some of your plans may not have worked as well. In this case, you must discover what went wrong. For example, did you take on too many activities at once? Were you too tired to stick to your plan? Was there enough time to do what you wanted? Did anyone keep you company or offer you support?

These and other such factors are capable of interfering with the best plans, and they may have been stumbling blocks for you too. But don't let discouragement get the upper hand. Learn from the errors. Plans can always be revised, and obstacles overcome. Hanging in there is far better than cheating yourself by giving up.

A practical suggestion is to *continually experiment* with changes in your exercise program. Look for new ways to make activity more feasible and personally enjoyable. Beginning at a relatively slow pace might be a change to consider. Plan to do some of your activities with friends or with a team. Join a health spa or your local "Y" where regular exercise is encouraged and your efforts rewarded. You might also consider reading up on physical fitness to discover new exercise options available to you.[4] Perhaps more frequent use of self-reward will get you off to a better start the next time.

After reconsidering your prior plan, list revisions you want to make to your list of planned activities (Table 6-4). Then put

---

[4]A useful reference on the subject is *Total Fitness in Thirty Minutes a Week* by Morehouse and Gross, listed in the reference section at the back of the book.

them into practice. Nothing is lost by continued experimentation, but a great deal can be lost by telling yourself you *can't* change—and the loss won't be in pounds.

MAINTAINING
A PHYSICAL ACTIVITY DIARY

Just as a diet diary (Chapter 5) provides immediate feedback on your eating habits, an activity diary can help you stay in touch with your activity habits. The logic is the same: When you observe or count behavior, you're in a better position to change it. You can count on that too.

A sample physical activity diary is shown in Table 6-5, along with the type of feedback it provides. We have constructed the diary as follows: Each small block in Column A represents ten minutes of activity. The letters inside the blocks correspond to the days of the week on which the activities are performed (M = Monday; T = Tuesday, and so forth). Column B shows the type of activity engaged in (outdoor walks, tennis, etc.); and Column C shows the number of calories expended per one minute of that activity. In Column D the number of ten-minute blocks of activity carried out during the entire week are tabulated, while Column E shows the total calories expended from each activity during that week. This Column-E value is obtained by multiplying Column C by Column D by the number 10 (C × D × 10 = calories per week).

For example, Bob's data are shown in Table 6-5. He recorded all the new and old physical activities he did during the week, one of which was taking daily walks around the neighborhood. On Monday he walked for a total of 30 minutes, on Tuesday for 10 minutes, on Wednesday for 30 minutes, and so on. Altogether he walked for about 120 minutes during the week, which, at 5.8 calories per minute, equals a caloric expenditure for this activity alone of 696 calories.

TABLE 6-5
Bob's Weekly Physical Activity Diary

(A) 10-minute blocks										(B) Activity	(C) Calories Per Minute	(D) # Blocks × 10	(E) Total Calories Expended
M F	M F	M	T	W	W	W	TH	TH	TH	#1 Walking outdoors	5.8	120	696
M T	W TH	F								#2 Work - walk up & down stairs		30	399
T	T	T	T	T	T					#3 Tennis	7	60	420
Su	Su	Su	Su	Su	Su	Su	Su	Su	Su	#4 Golf	5.5	120	660
Su	Su									Time spent walking & playing			

(1) Add right hand column to obtain total calories expended per week = <u>2175</u>

(2) Divide by 3500 calories to obtain pounds lost per week from physical activity =

<u>.62</u>

In addition to walking around the neighborhood, Bob made a commitment to use the stairs more often. He also made arrangements with his friend for a weekly tennis date, as well as taking up golf with his wife on the weekends. Altogether he was able to burn off 2175 calories for the week, more than half a pound of fat. If he maintains this program, he will lose over 32 pounds by the end of the year, just by exercising.

After revising your exercise program, you too might want to monitor your progress more closely by using a weekly physical activity diary. Cut the blank diaries in Appendix G along the dotted lines. Each week carry one with you or post it in a convenient spot (on your bathroom door, for example,) so you can record your physical activity each day. When you need additional blanks, make as many copies on a copy machine as you need. You may even devise an activity monitoring system you like better. If you continually monitor your activity program faithfully, you'll build new habits and enhance your commitment to change.

A weekly caloric intake, caloric expenditure, and weight loss graph has also been included for your convenience in Appendix H. If you find it helpful to see your progress, as most people do, then keep a weekly graph of your caloric intake, caloric expenditure, and weight. Graphing all three shows the relationship between them—the more you lower your intake and the more you exercise, the more weight you lose. Similarly, graphing quickly shows when problems begin.

Here's how to use the graph. Cut the graph along the dotted lines and tape it to a convenient spot, such as your bathroom or closet door. Write your daily caloric intake goal where it says "(Goal)" in the top panel, and write your weekly caloric expenditure goal where it says "(Goal)" in the middle panel. At the end of each week, (1) weigh yourself, (2) *total* your caloric expenditure for the week, and (3) total your daily caloric intake and divide by seven days to obtain your *average* intake for the week. Then record these numbers for the first week. Do this at the end of each week, and you can see your progress. Seeing your progress can be very rewarding. When you complete the graph (forty weeks), make a copy of the second blank graph and continue graphing your progress.

MUSCLE TONE EXERCISES

Besides exercising to increase energy expenditure and subsequently lose weight, you may also want to exercise to improve your muscle tone, or to shape and firm your body. *Muscle tone* exercises are particularly helpful to prevent the formation of hollow cheeks, soft arms, and a flabby stomach as you reduce. They are *not essential* for weight loss, but they can be a useful addition to any dietary plan. You may skip these exercises if you want.

The following series of basic muscle tone exercises can be done easily in the privacy of your home. Carried out three or four times a week for about ten minutes at a time, they won't take long to shape you up. If you would like additional information on muscle tone exercises and physical fitness, check the reference section at the back of the book.

1. WARM-UP
STRETCHING EXERCISES

High Stretch. As a preliminary warm-up exercise, stand up and slowly raise your arms as high as they can go. Try to stretch and reach the ceiling. Hold for five seconds. Relax and then repeat ten times.

Toe Touch. Another warm-up exercise is to stand with your legs about two feet apart, slowly bend over, and stretch your back and arms as far as you can. Relax, and then repeat ten times. When you start you will probably not be able to reach very far, but as you progress, you should eventually be able to touch your fingers to the floor.

2. FACIAL EXERCISES

To lessen pouches under the eyes and cheek hollows, close your eyes, and smile as hard as you can. Hold for ten seconds, and then relax. Repeat five times. To firm your jaw and chin, lean your head back as far as possible and slowly open and close your mouth ten times.

3. ARM EXERCISES

To firm up your upper arms, stand up straight with your legs about two feet apart. Hold a towel at both ends with your arms stretched out in front and pull firmly outward with both hands. Still holding onto the towel, slowly raise your arms above your head and then back to their original position. Repeat ten times. Extend your arms to the side and rotate them clockwide ten times, then counterclockwise ten times.

4. STOMACH AND ABDOMEN EXERCISES

Sit-Ups. To strengthen stomach muscles, lie on the floor and bend your knees slightly. Sit up and touch your toes with your hands and lie down again. Repeat ten times. *Leg Lifts.* Lie flat on the floor and slowly lift your legs about one foot off the floor, hold for five seconds and release. Repeat ten times.

5. LEG AND HIP EXERCISES

(a) To firm your thighs and hips try some knee bends. Stand with your feet apart and bend down to a high sitting position, then raise again. Repeat partial knee bends ten times. Do *not* go down to a full squat position, as this puts excessive stress on the knee joints. (b) For inner thighs and hips, lie on your left side with your right arm outstretched to steady the body. Holding your right leg straight, raise it as far as far as possible, then lower it. Repeat this ten times. Turn over and do the same exercise on the other side.

When you reduce your personal energy expenditure, you increase the probability of becoming obese. Physical activity is therefore essential in a total treatment program for weight loss.

The many benefits of including physical activities as part of your life include reducing your appetite, improving your shape, enhancing your health, making you feel better, making friends, helping the energy crisis—as well as the obvious benefit of burning off calories. After a candid look at your current physical activities, and suggestions for increasing them, we asked *you* to plan and implement your own physical activity program.

By now you have engaged in new physical activities, and achieved many little successes, and you should feel good about your progress and reward yourself accordingly. You probably have also experienced some setbacks. Since physical activity is not something you do once a week, but rather involves a whole approach to living a physically active, vigorous, zestful life, it takes time, patience and effort to develop these new patterns.

In the next chapter, you will see what you can do to enlist the aid of your family and friends in this effort.

Getting Support From Family and Friends

As you know, our personal relationships may help or hinder our weight loss efforts. You'll therefore be asked to collect and think about information on ways you can ask for assistance from your family and friends. In most cases you'll build on information you've already collected, but in some cases you'll be looking at behaviors and events for the first time. Each of the various assignments in this chapter may take about a week to complete, and all the assignments together may take several weeks. We recommend that you master all aspects of this chapter *before* moving ahead to the next chapter.

PERSONAL INTERACTIONS HELP AND HINDER WEIGHT LOSS

You might say, "It makes no difference what others do while I try to lose weight, because the success of my diet really depends on me." In a sense you're correct—what *you* do or not do will certainly determine whether you lose weight and keep it off. However, our behavior is strongly influenced by the actions of people around us. What others do, as well as the way they act toward us, influences our behavior. And this influence can make or break our efforts to change. A supportive social environment—people to talk with, to praise your successes, to listen to your sorrows—makes your efforts to *permanently* alter eating and exercise habits much easier. On the other hand, if the people around you criticize or undermine your attempts to lose weight, trying to change your eating habits can be a very frustrating and difficult experience. By the end of this chapter, perhaps you will better understand how your family and friends can influence your eating, and how you can enlist their *positive support.*

People can help you lose weight in many ways, just as they can hinder you in many ways. Table 7-1 contains a list of some these ways: Please add other examples based on your own experience.

IDENTIFY HELPERS
AND ASK FOR THEIR SUPPORT

How can you increase the helpful interactions while decreasing the hurtful ones? Begin by reviewing Table 3-4 in Chapter 3, in which you listed the important people in your life. Who are those people? How can they help? Select *two* people from your list. Choose persons you can trust and talk with, and who you feel comfortable about asking for assistance. In Table 7-2 write their names in the left-hand column and specify how you would like them to help in the right hand column. Ask these two persons for assistance and explain to them *in specific terms* what they can do. From then on they will be called your "helpers." Before reading any further, call or visit these two people and ask for their assistance.

TABLE 7-1

Ways That Help and Hinder Weight Loss

Ways that Help	*Ways that Hinder*
1. Remind you of your accomplishments in life.	1. Remind you of your previous weight failures.
2. Praise your new eating and exercise habits.	2. Criticize or ridicule your fatness.
3. Talk frequently about non-food activities.	3. Talk frequently about food.
4. Buy, prepare or serve you small quantities of low calorie foods.	4. Buy, prepare or serve you large quantities of high calorie foods.
5. Reward or praise you with appreciation instead of food.	5. Reward or praise you with food.
6. Listen to and support you when you are upset.	6. Ignore you when you are upset.
7. Avoid snacking in front of you.	7. Eat between meal snacks in front of you.
8. My mate is turned on to my thinner sexier appearance.	8. My mate is less interested in me sexually now that I am thinner.
9. _____	9. _____
10. _____	10. _____

What did the two people you selected say? Will they help you? If necessary, select somebody else and ask them for assistance too. Make sure you have at least two people you can count on for *long-term* help. Interact with them as you normally do, but also seek their assistance in the specific ways you have identified.

**IDENTIFY PEOPLE WHO HINDER
AND ASK THEM TO CHANGE**

Review again your list of important people in Chapter 3. This time select two people from the list whom you feel may hinder your efforts to lose weight, people who may, for exam-

TABLE 7-2

How I Would Like Others to Help

Name/Relationship	*How I Would Like Others to Help Me*
Examples:	
1. Lynn (spouse)	1. Go for a walk with me when I get edgy and am tempted to eat.
	2. Praise me regularly for changing my eating and exercise habits.
	3. Stop asking me to try rich desserts and candies.
2. Carol (good friend)	1. Talk with me when I'm upset and tempted to eat.
	2. Play tennis with me at least once every week.
	3. Encourage eating delicious, but low calorie foods.

Important people in your life

1. _____

   _____

1. _____
2. _____
3. _____

_____

_____

_____

2. _____

   _____

1. _____
2. _____
3. _____

_____

_____

_____

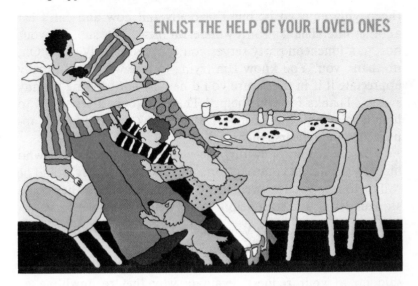

Courtesy of Dannon Milk Products. Used by permission.

ple, nag you about your weight, talk excessively about "fat" foods, or give you gifts of candy and other sweets. In Table 7–3, "People Who May Hinder My Weight Control Program," write down their names and how you would like them to change. Explain to these people that you are on a weight control program and that they could certainly help you by refraining from past practices. Be polite and positive. Tell them *exactly* how you would like them to change.

Asking people to change may sound simple, but it's often difficult to do. If you feel silly, concerned about starting a "fuss," or hesitant about asserting yourself, then try to rehearse what you want to say before a mirror or with your helper. For example, at an upcoming dinner party you know your hostess will offer you excessively large servings of food. You don't want to hurt her feelings, but you don't want to hurt your chances either! You might rehearse this situation by saying something like, "The food is really delicious and I have thoroughly enjoyed it, but I'm really full now and can't eat another bite. Thanks for a wonderful meal." Or suppose your host at a luncheon party serves you cookies. Simply say, "Oh, no thank you. You know I'm trying to lose weight. I'd really appreciate it if in the future you'd help by *not* offering me any sweets. Thanks for your help." These are only a few ways to handle common situations. Try to think of additional approaches and rehearse them.

Before reading any further, visit or call two people who hinder your weight control efforts and ask them if they would be willing to help you lose weight. Tell them exactly how they could stop hindering and start helping your weight control efforts.

What did they say? Were they a little surprised by your request? Are they willing to help? If they said yes, great! Tell them you appreciate their assistance. If they were ambivalent or said no to your request, evaluate why they're unwilling or unable to help.

Some people can be very insensitive to how difficult it is for you to control your weight. Others who are overweight themselves might feel jealous if you lose weight and they don't. You will probably have to learn either to assert yourself with these people or simply ignore them so they don't undermine your efforts. For example, it's perfectly appropriate for you to firmly ask the person who criticizes you to praise you instead for trying to become thin. Tell him or her that you would appreciate their spending more time *supporting* your weight control efforts than tearing them down. Explain how "flak" from others makes dieting much harder than it has to be. If the person really cares, he or she will probably try to change. However, you will have to give them time, patience, and lots of expression of appreciation. Their habits may be just as hard to change as your own.

For your overweight friends, explain to them the nature of this weight management program. You might even ask them to join you; if they accept, you can likely help each other lose weight. Consider forming a weight control group committed to

TABLE 7-3

People Who May Hinder My Weight Control Program

Name/ Relationship	Hinder	How I Would Like Them to Change
EXAMPLES 1. Martha (Mother-in-law)	Insists that I eat all the high calorie meals she prepares for me. If I don't, she feels that I don't love her.	1. Shows her "love" for me by helping me stay thin rather than helping me stay fat. 2. Prepare reasonable quantities of low calorie foods. 3. Let me serve my own food. 4. Accept my compliments about the quality, not the quantity of her cooking.
2. Steve (friend)	Serves fattening snacks at monthly poker party.	Offer non-fattening, or low calorie snacks at the monthly poker party.
People who *Hinder* 1. _____		1) _____ _____ 2) _____ _____ 3) _____ _____
2. _____		1) _____ _____ 2) _____ _____

going through these lessons, meeting regularly, and mutual help. Chapter 12 discusses additional ideas that can be used if you and another person want to lose weight together.

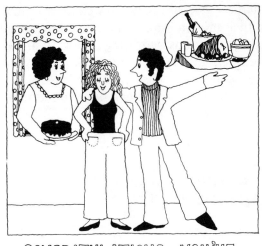

CONGRATULATIONS, YOU'VE MADE YOUR GOAL!

Courtesy of Dannon Milk Products. Used by permission.

Consider additional ways of tactfully asserting yourself so that others stop hindering you. There's nothing wrong with asserting yourself, as long as you don't infringe upon the rights of others. Sticking up for your right to become thin—even if that means saying no or requesting change from people you like—may seem awkward or uncomfortable at first. But it is *your right,* and in your own best interest to defend it. Some bestselling books have been written recently on tactful self-assertion.[1] If you haven't read them already, you might find them helpful and well worth the investment.

[1] For more information on how to be assertive see, Alberti & Emmons (1974); Bower and Bower (1976).

You should now be able to handle some of the personal interactions that hinder your weight loss. But a few people may really want to keep you overweight, as a way of controlling you and protecting themselves. Such persons give rise to a complicated situation, because they, as well as you, may not fully understand their motivation in wanting you to remain heavy. If you have these concerns, you might talk to the persons involved. You might also ask them to seek professional counseling. If these people still cause you problems, you might seek professional counseling so you can better understand why they bother you and how to deal with them.

REWARDING YOUR FAMILY AND FRIENDS FOR THEIR HELP

Sometimes you might be irritated because your friends neither recognize and praise your efforts nor your progress in weight control. Consider the other side of the coin. How often have you recognized or praised them for their help? Behavior is maintained largely by the consequences it produces. If you want their help, show them your respect and appreciation when it occurs. You should try to express this warmly and directly, for it will do little good if it is not understood. Don't make the common mistake of assuming they'll realize your appreciation. Let them know. Try saying, "Thank you, Mary, for not offering me sweets at the party," or "Thanks, Bill, for listening to me when I was upset and about to go on a food binge." Even send little thank-you notes or a small gift to those who help you a lot. Experiment with whatever you think is an appropriate way of showing your appreciation. *Develop ways of helping them help you.*

If you continue to work with the important people in your life, they will stop hindering and start helping your weight control efforts. Some of your efforts will pay off immediately while others may not. You should therefore reward yourself for the ones that work and reconsider the ones that do not. Trial and error will eventually lead to trial and success. Propose different ways of interacting with these people, and keep trying until you establish healthy, positive ways of mutual influence.

After establishing your dietary tools and your relationships with helpers, you are ready to concentrate on the next task, which is managing your food—the subject of the following chapter.

8

Managing Food: How to Buy, Store, Clean-Up, Prepare, Serve, Eat, and Snack on Food

As you learned in Chapter 2, certain cues and situations in your environment influence much of your eating behavior, including what, when, and how much you eat each day. In our mass-media society, you are literally bombarded with cues to "eat, eat, eat." The next time you watch television, for example, count the number of times and ways you are urged to eat candy or drink soda pop. Even work routines can condition you to eat in certain situations and not in others. For example, a coffee-break may mean buying a doughnut or candy bar—even though you had a hearty breakfast just two hours before! Similarly, getting ready to watch a favorite soap opera or read a thrilling novel may be a cue to raid the refrigerator. On the other hand, working in the garden, cleaning the house, or help-ing the kids with their homework may almost never be ac-companied by eating.

The process in which certain situations set the stage for behavior, or serve as a cue to do something is technically called the *stimulus control of behavior.* All this phrase means is that you are a *discriminating* person; that is, you learn to do things under certain conditions but not under others. How stimulus control is learned is not fully understood, but apparently, we learn to associate certain situational cues with certain behavior, and certain resultant consequences. Each time the behavior is followed by the reinforcing consequence, the cue influences our behavior a little more.

For overweight people, stimulus or *situational control* is very important. Because of conditioned eating responses to these food cues, eating occurs too often in too many situations. Therefore in certain situations—such as a tantalizing food advertisement, a pastry shop, loneliness or boredom—the urge to eat may be irresistible. The secret to effective situational management is to eliminate wherever possible these food cues so as to eliminate the urge to eat. Some cues cannot be eliminated entirely so the secret here is to substitute new behaviors for eating. In both cases, you are practicing effective self-management; that is, you are learning to act in ways that will help you control unnecessary eating.

The act of eating itself is the final link in a long chain of behaviors. The first link may be buying the food, the second storing it, the third link preparing it, the fourth serving it, and the fifth link eating it. In this chapter we focus on a careful analysis of the different behaviors within this chain and pro-pose practical methods to control them. If the early links are ef-fectively managed, then the final link, eating, can be more easi-ly controlled.

HOW DO YOU MANAGE FOOD?

How do you presently manage food? Answering the questions in Table 8-1 will help you assess these habits quickly and honestly. You may find it difficult to categorize your eating habits since they sometimes vary from meal to meal and day to day. However, do your best and write the letter (a), (b) or (c) in the column on the right that seems *most* representative of your habits. Then add up the number of (c) and (b) responses. If you have sixteen or more, you already have a good set of food management behaviors. Congratulations! If you have less than sixteen, you need to make some changes.

TABLE 8-1
My Current Food Management Behaviors

Directions: Write the letter (a), (b), or (c) in the column that most represents your food habits.

(a) (b) (c)

I. *Buying Food*
1. Do you usually go to the grocery store (a) without a written food list, (b) with some ideas in your head about what to buy (but no list), (c) with a written food list?
2. Do you usually buy (a) whatever meets your fancy in the aisles and on the shelves, (b) more than you originally had on your list, (c) from your food list only?
3. Do you usually shop (a) when you are hungry, (b) whenever you need to, (c) when you are not hungry?
4. Do you usually purchase (a) unnecessary quantities of most foods, (b) unnecessary quantities of some food, (c) only moderate quantities of food?
5. Do you buy mostly (a) high-calorie foods, (b) a combination of high- and low-calorie foods, or (c) low-calorie, nutritious foods?

Table 8–1 (*cont.*)

II. *Storing Food*
1. Do you usually store food in (a) transparent, accessible containers in the refrigerator, (b) whatever is handy, or (c) in opaque, (non-see-through), difficult-to-reach containers in the refrigerator? _____
2. Do you usually store food in (a) transparent, easy-to-reach containers in the cupboards, (b) whatever is handy, or (c) in opaque, difficult to reach containers in the cupboards. _____
3. Do you (a) usually leave food on the kitchen countertop, in the living room, or in the TV room, (b) sometimes leave food on the kitchen countertop, in the living room, or in the TV room, or (c) almost never leave food on the kitchen countertop, in the living room, or in the TV room? _____

III. *Preparing Food*
1. (a) Do others usually prepare your food, or (b) do you usually prepare your own food? _____
2. Do you (or others) usually prepare (a) high calorie meals or (b) low-calorie meals? _____
3. Do you (or others) usually prepare (a) quantities of food for more than one helping or (b) quantities sufficient for only *one* helping? _____

IV. *Serving Food*
1. (a) Do others usually serve your food, or (b) do you usually serve your own food? _____
2. Do you usually serve (a) more than you need, or (b) a moderate portion? _____
3. Do you usually serve yourself (a) second portions or (b) only one portion? _____
4. Do you usually (a) put bowls or food containers on the table or (b) leave them in the kitchen? _____

V. *Eating*
1. Do you put (a) a large or (b) a small quantity of food on your spoon or fork? _____
2. Do you chew your food (a) rapidly or (b) slowly? _____
3. Do you (a) put one bite of food after another into your mouth or (b) wait between bites? _____

Table 8–1 (*Cont.*)

    4. Do you (a) eat so fast you don't have time to enjoy
       your food or (b) do you eat slowly enough to enjoy it
       thoroughly?   _____
    5. Do you (a) eat all the food in front of you or (b) stop
       eating when you're full even though there's food on
       your plate?   _____

  VI. *Cleaning-Up*
    1. After eating do you (a) sit around or (b) leave the
       table?   _____
    2. After finishing the main dish do you (a) leave the
       leftovers on the table or (b) clear the table before
       having a cup of coffee or tea?   _____

 VII. *Snacking*
    1. Do you snack (a) frequently (say, more than three
       times daily) or (b) occasionally?   _____
    2. Do you snack (a) large quantities of food (e.g., a
       sandwich and a piece of cake) or (b) small quantities
       of food?   _____
    3. Do you snack (a) high-calorie foods (e.g., cookies)
       or (b) low-calorie foods (e.g., celery and carrots)?   _____

                          Total number (a) responses   _____

                          Total number (b) responses   _____

                          Total number (c) responses   _____

SOME GOOD WAYS TO MANAGE FOOD

Evidence from research and clinical experience suggests
the following good food management tips. They are broken
down according to each of the links in the chain of food consumption: buying, storing, preparing, serving, eating, cleaning-
up, and snacking.

I. BUYING FOOD

1. Prepare a low-calorie, balanced food list.

2. Shop from your food list only. In an effort to stimulate your buying impulse, marketing research has shown store keepers how to display their food attractively to get you to buy more than you need. Buying from your list is sensible counter-control.

3. Shop when you're *not* hungry. The hungrier you are, the more likely you are to buy food impulsively. Go shopping *after* you've eaten a meal rather than before. Drink a glass of water or dietetic soda before shopping if you are beginning to feel hungry.

4. Buy only what you need to eat. If there is no extra food in the house, you can't eat it.

5. Buy low-calorie, high-nutrition, and tasty foods. Chapter 5 discussed the nutritional and caloric value of foods. Buy foods that are low in calorie but still satisfying to your taste. Experiment, try different foods the next time you shop.

II. STORING FOOD

1. Store food in opaque, inaccessible containers in the refrigerator or cupboards. If you can't see them everytime you open the refrigerator or cupboard door, or if you have to reach back into inaccessible places, you'll be less tempted to eat.

2. Remove all food from the living room, TV room, and the kitchen countertops. People can eat large quantities of food while watching TV without realizing how much they

have eaten. Take all food out of the living room and away from the TV. Food in plain sight is often eaten; food out of sight is often out of mind.

III. PREPARING FOOD

1. Prepare low-calorie, high-nutrition meals. You might review the section in Chapter 5 that dealt with calorie intake and diets for some specific ideas.
2. Prepare moderate quantities only, enough for a *single* serving to yourself and each person present.
3. Don't nibble while preparing the food. Consuming your meal before you sit down to eat is easy. If you must have food in your mouth while preparing, chew on a piece of celery, or a piece of sugarless gum.
4. Take responsibility for the preparation of your food. And if you prepare your own food, take steps to prepare it properly. If others prepare your meals for you, ask them politely to prepare your food in accordance with the suggestions we have given. If extra quantities of food are *not* prepared, they will not be around to eat.

IV. SERVING FOOD

1. Serve just enough food to meet your caloric needs for that meal. Typically this is a small or medium helping.
2. Don't go back for seconds.
3. Don't serve "family style"; that is, leave large bowls of food on the table. Instead, put food on a plate and leave the bowl in the kitchen.

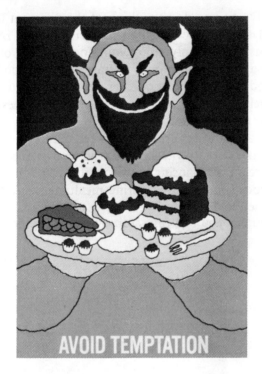

Courtesy of Dannon Milk Products. Used by permission.

V. EATING

Eating should be a healthy, enjoyable experience. However, for the overweight it is often neither. Many overweight people eat so fast, their bodies don't have time to tell them when to stop eating, not do their minds have a chance to enjoy the food. Slow down the chewing action of your jaws to about two bites per second, and you will eat less food while enjoying it more. Put a small quantity of food on your spoon or fork (there's no need to overload your utensils) and chew the food slowly. As you do this, think of the different tastes, textures, and smells of each small morsel you eat. By chewing slower you will not only enjoy your food more, you will also allow the saliva in your mouth to start digesting food so it will be absorbed into your body quicker. In this way you will reduce the time delay between eating and a sense of fullness, without overeating in the process.

Pause about thirty seconds between each bite of food you take. Put your fork down, think of what you have eaten, talk to someone, relax. By pausing between bites you will also be able to enjoy social interactions during mealtime, as well as allow your stomach to digest the food you've consumed.

As soon as you feel full, stop eating. Stopping may sound

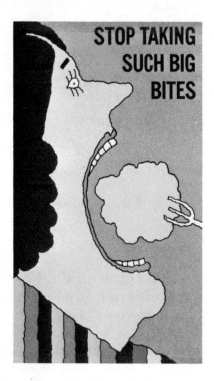

Courtesy of Dannon Milk Products. Used by permission.

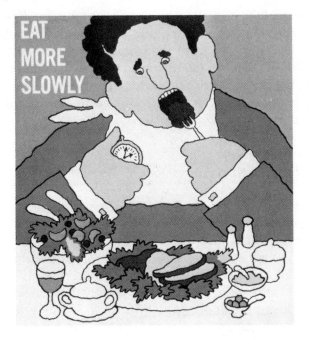

Courtesy of Dannon Milk Products. Used by permission.

simple, but often it's not. If you eat big bites quickly, your body cannot tell you to stop eating until after you have passed the full level and have become overly stuffed. The body needs several minutes to realize it's had enough; sometimes the delay is ten to fifteen minutes or more. Focus on your body, slow down your eating, enjoy what you eat, and when you feel full—stop! Let your body help you experience the pleasure of eating by taking it slow and easy.

VI. CLEANING-UP

Clear the table immediately after completing the main dish. If you enjoy sitting at the table after eating to talk with others or to have a cup of coffee, do so and enjoy yourself. But clean the table first. If there is food on the table you'll probably nibble; and soon you may nibble a second and third helping of food. Clear the food from the plates and store it or throw it away. No, discarding food is not a mortal sin; why not serve smaller portions in the first place. If it's inconvenient to clear the table immediately, then leave it; go to another room for your conversation or cup of coffee.

VII. SNACKING

We all like to snack. But don't let snacking become your main source of calories. On the contrary, avoid the trap of trying never to snack and then experiencing failure. If you find yourself hungry at midmorning, maybe you missed your breakfast or failed to get enough protein at breakfast. If so, eat a breakfast with more protein and eliminate your snack. By eating a high-protein breakfast (fifteen to twenty grams), you can reduce hunger and change snacking habits more easily.

Are your present snacks high-calorie foods—candy, cake, cookies? Consider low-calorie snacks such as celery, carrots, popcorn, oranges, pears, apples, pickles, cauliflower, raw vegetables. Buy *small* quantities of *low*-calorie snacks and have them available when you take a snack break.

YOUR FOOD MANAGEMENT PROGRAM

Evaluate your current eating behaviors. In the left-hand column of Table 8-2, "My Food Management Program," write down all the behaviors for which you scored (a) in Table

TABLE 8-2
My Food Management Program

Troublesome Behaviors (Add specific examples)	Proposed Changes
Example *Buying Food* *I shop for food without a written list.*	*Prepare a written food list before going to the grocery store and buy only what is on it.*

I. Buying Food

II. Storing Food

III. Preparing Food

IV. Serving Food

V. Eating Food

VI. Cleaning-Up

VII. Snacking

8-1. Since the (a) categories represent behavior that leads to excessive intake, these are the ones that need changing. Though changing all these behaviors at once is difficult, you must eventually try to change as many of them as you can, because they often lead to uncontrolled eating. Think about them for awhile and then propose alternative positive behaviors that *you can realistically fit into your life style.* Try focusing on those food habits that lead to extra fattening calories for you. Think of the food management tips suggested earlier and add your own as well. Write these alternatives under the column entitled, "Proposed Changes," of your food management program.

Your final task for this chapter is to implement your proposed changes one at a time. In order to avoid taking on too much too soon, we suggest you master each proposed change before going on to the next one. And master these changes before going on to the next chapter. Complete mastery may take several weeks, to several months. Don't get discouraged—your old food habits have had years of practice; much time and effort will be needed to establish your new ones.

REVIEW

How have you been doing since completing some of your proposed changes? Were some of your new behaviors easy to implement? If so, great! Congratulate yourself for the progress you've made and keep up the good work. Other changes may have given you some trouble. Consider what went wrong: Were they unrealistic proposals? Were certain old habits more difficult to change than you thought? Were there too many changes to implement at one time? Maybe you found it hard to alter your shopping habits suddenly, or you were overly ambitious in thinking that you could limit your meals to a single helping of food? That's okay. Try proposing a new plan of action to correct these obstacles and test it out. You don't have to change every habit, but you do have to change those habits that lead to excessive eating. Continue to monitor your progress and reinforce yourself for doing a good job. With effort and patience you will eventually develop a new set of eating habits essential for permanent weight control.

One habit in particular may be troubling you. Very often, many people resort to eating when upset, bored, or angry. Perhaps in the next chapter, we can help you deal with your feelings without consuming unnecessary food.

9

Learning To Handle Your Feelings Without Eating

To be human is to experience many different feelings and moods. We all experience moments of joy and sadness, of boundless energy and complete exhaustion, of relaxation and anxiety. Sometimes we feel fulfilled, other times bored, or perhaps angry and frustrated. Living a good life involves learning to understand, accept, and handle our feelings. We all have learned different ways to handle various feelings, some healthier ways than others.

Almost everyone, when they encounter moments of exhaustion, anxiety, boredom, loneliness, or anger handle those feelings by eating. Eating can comfort us when we're upset. People of normal weight *occasionally* comfort themselves by eating, while overweight people *frequently* handle their unhappy feelings by eating. Persons without weight problems have

165

learned non-eating alternatives to reduce negative feelings. Some of these alternatives have problems associated with them too—such as drugs, alcohol, or smoking—But if our focus is on helping you develop positive, healthy, and nonfattening ways to deal with certain feelings, then the first step is properly identifying your feelings.

COMMON FEELINGS
THAT GIVES US DIFFICULTY

1. *Tiredness* involves feelings of either physical, mental, or emotional fatigue, or exhaustion. You feel too tired to do anything. This feeling is often experienced during or after a hard day's work at the office or after a day with the kids. A common way of handling this feeling is to rest. Another is to take a food break—to sit and consume calories by drinking and eating.

2. *Anxiety* involves fear, restlessness, agitation, sweating palms, tightened muscles. Anxiety is frequently experienced when you anticipate a threat to your well-being, whether real or imagined. For example, you may not be sure whether the visit with your in-laws will work out, whether you'll be promoted in your job, whether your child will recover from an illness, or whether your marriage will continue. Again, a common response to anxiety is nervous eating. An overweight person often attempts to alleviate his anxiety by eating, and soothing himself with food.[1]

3. *Boredom* involves thinking you have nothing you need or want to do. Boredom is often experienced by housewives who, after sending their children to school and completing their house chores, find themselves with nothing to do. Even though

[1]See G. Rosen, *Don't Be Afraid* for ways to reduce fears and anxieties.

you may not be hungry, the buying, preparing, and eating of food are at least doing something.

4. *Loneliness* involves the feeling of having no intimate relationships, close friends, or companions to do things with. Loneliness is often experienced by people who have difficulty initiating or maintaining friendships.

5. *Anger* involves feelings of resentment, bitterness, jealousy, indignation, and frustration. These feelings often occur when you are prevented from obtaining a goal you desire. For example, you may have requested a vacation at a specific time and your boss turned you down. You then become angry with him. Or you may expect your spouse home on time for dinner, but he arrives home an hour late without calling you in advance. While there are many different ways of reducing anger, one way is to soothe it by eating.

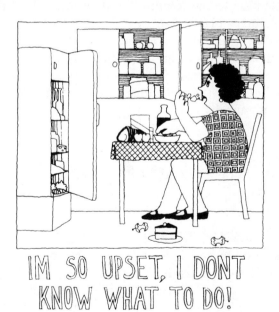

IM SO UPSET, I DONT KNOW WHAT TO DO!

Courtesy of Dannon Milk Products. Used by permission.

FEELINGS AND YOUR TYPICAL
RESPONSES TO THEM

Identifying feelings can be difficult because many of us have learned to repress them. Our society and culture teaches us to submerge our feelings, especially negative feelings, such as anger, resentment, anxiety, and loneliness. Unfortunately, repressing feelings over the long run causes more harm than good. Becoming aware of your feelings and learning to accept them, though a difficult step, is an important one if you are to control your weight successfully.

Look over your Eating Diary from Chapter 3, paying particular attention to the column that describes your feelings. In the sample diary (Table 3–6), excessive eating occurred when the person was tired, angry, or bored. Write *your* common feelings on "Your Feelings Chart" (Table 9–1) and jot down your typical responses to these feelings under the column "Typical Response." Leave the remaining column blank for now. Be honest with yourself!

SOME NON-WEIGHTY ALTERNATIVES
TO EATING

As mentioned earlier, both normal-weight and overweight people use food to handle their feelings, but obese people tend to use food more frequently. Therefore the goals of this lesson are to practice and increase alternative (*non*-eating) ways to handle your feelings. In the following paragraphs are a number of suggestions for you to consider. At the end of this chapter you will be asked to select some of them to practice on your own.

TABLE 9–1
Your Feelings Chart

Your Feelings (Add Specific Examples)	Your Typical Response	Your Proposed Alternatives
EXAMPLE: Tiredness I'm usually burned out by mid-afternoon after taking care of the kids all day.	Snack on whatever's available. It seems to pick me up.	Rest quietly for 15 minutes with only a cup of coffee.
1. Tiredness		
2. Anxiety		
3. Boredom		
4. Loneliness		
5. Anger		

1. NAPPING AND SLEEPING

If you're tired during the day, take a nap break rather than a food break. You'll feel better and consume *no* calories. You may say you're unable to nap or you can't find a quiet spot during the daytime. However, by trying a little harder most people can find a quiet spot to nap or simply to sit and rest for awhile.

If you're unable to nap or are still tired afterward, consider going to bed earlier. The extra sleep will make you feel better, and again you consume *no* calories while sleeping. You may have to take a careful look at how you spend your evenings, especially after 9 or 10 P.M. Getting to bed earlier might really make a difference.[2] Sleeping demonstrates that you can go for about eight hours *without eating*.

2. PHYSICAL ACTIVITY

The advantages of physical activity have already been discussed. In addition to burning off calories, physical activity can relax you, reduce tension, lessen boredom, curb anger, and reduce "nervous" hunger. You should therefore feel better if you've practiced the physical activity program in Chapter 6.

Are there other physical activities you can do to help you manage your feelings more effectively? Yes! For example, try taking a brisk walk or bike ride the next time you become anxious or angry. Join a gym club. Take part in community recreational activities. Spend time gardening or housecleaning, mowing the lawn, rearranging furniture, walking the dog, hitting some tennis or golf balls—rather than "hitting" the refrigerator. You can at the same time control emotional reactions and burn off calories with physical activity.

[2]Coates and Thoresen (*How To Sleep Better*) offer several things you can do to feel more rested and relaxed during the day.

3. PHYSICAL RELAXATION ACTIVITIES

Hot Bath, Shower or Sauna.   If you find yourself tired, anxious, or angry, try taking a hot bath, a shower, or a sauna. Even sitting in a chair with your legs elevated and a cool cloth on your face can be very relaxing.

Muscle Relaxation.   Alternately tensing and releasing various muscle groups can also reduce bodily tension. Practice the following exercises while sitting in a comfortable chair or lying down. Clench both of your fists as tightly as you can and carefully notice the tension in them. Remember, however, not to overdo it: Clench them just tightly enough to feel the tension. Now relax both fists and feel the tension run out and the relaxation flow in. Tighten both arms as tightly as you can— hold them that way for about five seconds and feel the tension. Now let go and feel the tension disappear and the relaxation appear. You are very gradually becoming relaxed. Tighten your shoulder and neck muscles, tighter and tighter—feel the tension. Now, letting loose, feel yourself more and more relaxed. Take a slow, deep breath, hold the air in your lungs as long as you can. Now exhale slowly . . . slowly . . . as you become more calm and relaxed. Continue tightening, holding, and then relaxing other groups of muscles in your body—head, stomach, legs—until all your muscles are relaxed. When you become anxious or upset, practice these exercises in a quiet place at work or at home instead of eating.[3]

4. CALL OR VISIT FRIENDS

Put Chapter 7, which dealth with enlisting the support of friends, to good use in handling your feelings. When you feel

[3]See Rosen, *Don't Be Afraid,* for detailed instructions on muscle relaxation skills.

uptight, anxious, lonely, or bored call or visit a helping friend. Better yet, keep a list of several friends to contact: In case one is not home, you'll have others to call. Remember to thank them for helping you—but don't let them try to make you feel better by offering you fattening foods!

5. INSTANT ACTIVITIES

Develop a list of "instant" non-eating activities you can do in place of eating, that is, things you can do without advance notice. If you become upset and feel like eating, go to a movie, shop for clothes, visit a museum, take a brisk walk, tour a zoo, read a fun book, do whatever turns you on. Develop a list of activities you can do at a moment's notice, with little or no pre-planning. (A trip to the South Seas might be great but not readily available.) Choose things you really enjoy doing, but please don't bring or buy food while doing it. Since you are giving up food that is "important" to you, now is the time to indulge in non-food activities that you enjoy.

6. LONG-TERM HOBBIES AND SOCIAL SERVICE ACTIVITIES

If you find yourself feeling generally bored or unfulfilled, consider getting involved in some long-term hobbies, social activities, or community service projects. You might say, "I don't have time for that," but have you ever tried to make time? After all, it takes time to sit and eat too.

There are numerous hobbies you might take up. What do you like to do? Crafts, arts, travel, reading, cultural activities are all available to you. Call the Parks and Recreation Center in your area; they can tell you what activities are available. There

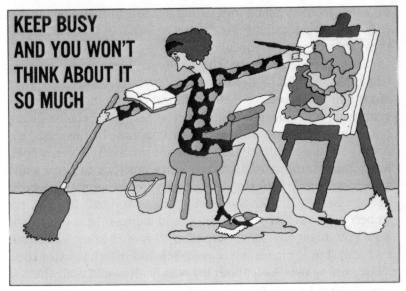

KEEP BUSY
AND YOU WON'T
THINK ABOUT IT
SO MUCH

Courtesy of Dannon Milk Products. Used by permission.

are all sorts of social clubs from dance to stamp collecting, from gardening to ski clubs. There are also many interesting community service projects that need volunteer help: The United Way, March of Dimes, conservation groups, environmental protection associations, individual tutoring projects in hospitals and schools—others are crying for your help. In the process of helping others you may find greater fulfillment and a bit more happiness; at the same time you won't be eating, and gaining weight.

7. EXPRESS YOUR ANGER

If you feel angry, become aware of it and try to understand the events that led up to it. You may have done something that made you feel angry toward yourself. While denying your anger by going to the kitchen and eating is easy, in the long run becoming aware of conditions that set you off and then changing them are much more helpful responses.

If you become angry with someone, contact one of your helpers to tell him or her how angry you are. Expressing your anger will make you feel better without consuming calories. By expressing and understanding your anger, you become aware that some people do things that irritate you. In this case, express your anger directly to the people involved. For example, Mary may continually offer you extra portions of food while criticizing people for being fat. Your typical response may be to become upset with her and then go home and eat. Instead, try to become aware of your feelings and express them directly to her. You might say something like, "Mary, I know you mean no harm, but it makes me upset when you offer me extra food while putting me down about my weight. It would really help if you wouldn't offer me any food." Identify what makes you angry and, where appropriate, talk it over with the person involved.

The discussion in Chapter 7 about assertive training and dealing with others is also relevant in regard to expressing your feelings appropriately.[4]

DEVELOP NON-FATTENING WAYS TO HANDLE YOUR FEELINGS

After assessing your feelings and your typical eating responses to them, and after considering the presentation of some non-weighty alternatives to eating, propose specific, concrete,

[4]See the books by Alberti and Emmons (1974) and Bower and Bower (1976) for more information on assertive training and expressing your feelings.

non-fattening alternative ways to handle your feelings. Use any of our suggestions that seem helpful to you, and add your own as well. Now write all your proposed changes on Your Feeling Chart (Table 9–1).

Your next, and most difficult, task is to implement each of these proposed changes. Approach this task in the same way you have approached previous chapter goals. Take one change at a time and implement it for one or two weeks. Then evaluate what happened. If it was successful, reward yourself. If it was not successful, examine what happened: Was the standard unrealistic? Did you practice or sufficiently rehearse the behavior before implementing it? Did you have the support of family or friends? Modify your proposal and try again. The important thing is to master each proposed change before going on to the next one. Since some proposed changes are naturally easier to implement than others, do the easier one first to get a taste of success before tackling the more difficult feelings.

A word of caution is needed: Everyone experiences negative feelings. And we have tried to assist you in becoming more aware of these feelings and in developing non-fattening, healthy alternative ways to deal with them. But if anxiety, loneliness, or anger occur with great intensity and high frequency, they may be signs of more serious personal problems. In this case, it is advisable to consult a psychologist or your family physician for professional counseling.

If you're like most people, however, you deal with the same special eating problems that everyone else does. In the next chapter, we'll go into these problems in detail.

10

Progressing Toward Long-Range Goals: It Takes Time and Effort

Congratulations upon completing the previous chapters. You've made great strides toward learning new life long habits to control your weight. But because your old habits took many years to develop, learning new ones permanently will take still more work. If you still have difficulty in following some of the weight control lessons, turn back to the chapter that dealt with the problem: Reread, review, and do the chapter again until you have completely mastered the lesson.

This chapter discusses methods of handling special eating situations as well as the old problem of the weight plateau.

HANDLING SPECIAL EATING SITUATIONS

Dieting is hard work, and handling certain dieting situations can be particularly difficult. Such situations include drinking certain beverages between meals, going to dinner parties, eating at restaurants or on vacations, having big holiday meals, watching a skinny spouse always eating, or paying premium prices for diet foods in inflationary times. Although such situations are common stumbling blocks for people trying to lose weight, they need not be your Achilles heel.

In general, you can handle all these special situations by applying the principles and lessons discussed in the previous chapters. Also, you must learn to *plan ahead*. So when you know you'll be going to a dinner party or to a choice restaurant, eat a little less in the morning and the next day, and exercise a little more to compensate for the meal. Let's examine some ways to deal with special situations based on ideas you have already received.

DRINKING

Some people mistakenly believe that because they are drinking liquids, they are taking in very few or no calories, which is certainly true for water, coffee, and tea—but that's about all. If you don't believe that, check the caloric values in Table 10-1.

The calories from a single drink may not seem like much, but they accumulate each day. For example, a secretary who has a regular mid-morning and mid-afternoon coke break five days a week consumes 75,400 calories a year due to these breaks alone: 145 calories per 12-oz. coke × 10 per week × 52 weeks = 75,400. The salesman who has two beers or martinis nightly to relax after a hard day's work also takes in about the same number of calories. At 3,500 calories per pound, that figure is the equivalent of 21 pounds of fat a year! If the secretary switched to tea or coffee (without cream and sugar) or to sugar-free carbonated beverages, she could lose up to 21 pounds per year. And if the salesman used relaxation exercises, took a walk, or played tennis to unwind, he could lose the same amount.

Let's say your problem begins when you go to a cocktail

TABLE 10-1

Caloric Value of Common Beverages

	Calories
Carbonated Beverages	
Cola-type, 12-oz. can or bottle	145
Fruit Flavors, 12-oz. can or bottle	170
Table Wines	
Chablis, Sauterne, and the like, 6-oz. glass	150
Beer	
12-oz. can or bottle	150
Whisky, Gin, Rum, Vodka, Scotch	
90 proof, 1½-oz. jigger	110
Cocktails	
Martini	140
Brandy Alexander	225

party or lounge. If you enjoy an alcoholic drink, we're not suggesting that you abstain or that you reduce the pleasure you derive; we're only suggesting that you try to reduce the caloric cost of drinking. Try ordering lower-calorie drinks, such as dry wines rather than beer, or whiskey on the rocks instead of a Brandy Alexander. Mix drinks with sugar-free carbonated beverages. Limit yourself to one or two drinks. Sip them slowly; don't gulp them down. In the long run you'll save not only calories but money as well.[1]

EATING OUT

Eating at a luncheon with neighbors, a dinner party given by a friend, or a restaurant all pose special problems. The routine of your diet at home is disrupted when you eat out. However, many of the same basic food principles you use at home still apply and you will find them helpful in controlling your intake if you keep them in mind.

[1]If you have trouble limiting your drinking, see Miller and Munoz, *How to Control Your drinking.*

For example, when at a restaurant, you can easily order clear soups (such as consomme), fresh salads (without dressing or oil and vinegar), lean meats, fish, vegetables, sugar-free coffee or tea. No law states that you must order such *high-calorie* foods as creamed soups, breaded and fried meats, french fried potatoes, milk shakes, bread, and desserts. Many low-calorie, tasty dishes are usually available. If your favorite restaurant doesn't have any low-calorie dishes, find another one that does.

If you are eating at a luncheon, dinner party, or picnic, serve yourself *small* quantities of low-calorie foods. Others may expect you to eat a lot of whatever's available, but, again, no law says you must. By serving yourself you will avoid having others put too much food on your plate.

Whether you're at a restaurant or someone's home, always try to eat slowly. Take small bites of food; chew them slowly. Put your fork down between bites and talk to the people around you. When you begin to feel full, stop eating, even if there is still food on your plate. Enjoy both your food and your company.

After you've finished eating, ask the waiter to clear the table so you will not sit there nibbling. If your hostess doesn't clear the table immediately, offer to do it for her. You will be helping not only her but yourself as well.

Another problem situation, as previously noted, is when your hostess offers you second helpings or a big dessert. Though the situation is sensitive, nothing is wrong with a polite refusal. If you assert yourself by saying, "No thank you. The food was delicious but I'm on a diet and have had enough," she'll probably understand and not be offended.

HOLIDAYS AND VACATIONS

Thanksgiving, New Year's, birthdays, anniversaries, and other special occasions are often celebrated with large meals. They are meant to be joyous occasions and they should be. By planning ahead for these events, however, you need not gain weight. Because you know when to expect holidays you can't excuse bad eating habits by saying, "There wasn't time to plan ahead." Whenever you expect to eat a *little* more, try compensating for your overindulgence by reducing your caloric intake and/or by increasing your caloric expenditure. Do this a day or two before and after the holiday celebration. In this way you can control you weight, as well as enjoy the festivities.

Vacations also represent a break in your regular work and home routine, but they need not upset your diet if you apply the principles and suggestions already presented. Plan a relaxing vacation that includes many physical activities such as swimming, tennis, or touring on foot. If you should happen to eat more food than you need, compensate for it by increasing your exercise or eating less at the next meal.

YOUR SKINNY SPOUSE OR FRIENDS ARE ALWAYS EATING

Sometimes you may feel discouraged because your friends *seem* to eat more than you but never gain weight. The important word in the last sentence is "seems." You must admit your perceptions of other people are sometimes inaccurate. For example, others may eat more than you when you see them, but they don't nibble or go on food binges at other times. They don't gain weight probably because they consume *fewer calories overall* than you think. If you're really concerned about this, ask the person to keep an eating diary for one week: If he or she agrees you can simply add up the calories and compare them with yours.

Even if you find that the normal-weight person consistently eats more than you, he or she may maintain a good weight because of greater physical activity or a higher basal metabolism. One way or the other, they burn off what they take in, thus maintaining a balance between caloric intake and ex-

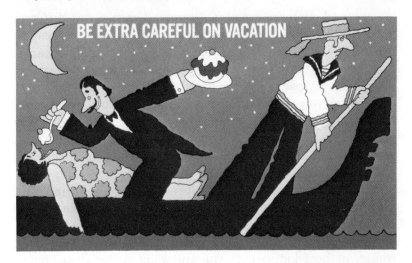

BE EXTRA CAREFUL ON VACATION

Courtesy of Dannon Milk Products. Used by permission.

penditure. Everyone has a balance point. If you remember there are individual differences, you may not feel so bad the next time you compare yourself with others. Besides, making comparisons will *not* help *you* lose weight.

DIETING AND THE RISING COST OF FOOD

With the rising cost of food, you may be tempted to rationalize excessive eating by saying you can't afford to stay on a diet. After all, special diet foods do cost quite a bit. Although the rising cost of food makes balancing a budget more and more difficult, you can do a number of things to cut calories *and* cost without sacrificing a balanced diet.

First, reduce the quantity of food you buy and you will *also reduce costs;* buy only as much food as you need to meet your caloric and nutritional requirements.

Second, become a smart shopper. Learn about different types of low-calorie, low-cost, high-nutrition foods. Instead of processed foods, buy fresh foods which are generally cheaper. For the same reason, try cooking more with basic ingredients instead of pre-packaged, prepared foods. Buy low-cost, low-calorie, raw vegetables and fruits: Vegetables such as broccoli, brussel sprouts, cabbage, cauliflower, celery, cucumber, green beans, greens, lettuce, mushrooms, okra, peppers, sauerkraut, summer squash are all excellent choices. Many of them taste good raw and make nice snacks.

Third, vary your diet with leaner meats, fowl, and fish. Stop buying expensive marbled (that is, fatty and high-calorie) steaks and switch to lean flank and round steaks instead. Experiment also with less popular meats such as pot roast, ground round, or beef kidneys. If you still want prime steak, buy a smaller portion and supplement it with high protein dairy products, such as low-fat cottage cheese. Poultry—chicken, turkey, and duck—are all high in protein and typically less expensive than beef, and it can be prepared in many low-calorie ways. Seafood and shellfish too are excellent sources of protein while usually low in calories. Favorites like salmon or lobster are expensive, but items such as perch and mussels are less expensive.

Finally, many low-calorie recipes are available for preparing almost any food you buy, expensive or not. A list of such recipes can be found in Appendix C, and several good low-calorie cookbooks can be found in the references.

OVERCOMING YOUR DIFFICULT
EATING SITUATIONS

Although people trying to diet have many difficult eating situations in common, very often one person's weakness may be another person's strength. Since only you know which situations prey on your weaknesses, only you can pinpoint these situations, propose solutions, implement the proposals, and then evaluate what happened.

The best approach is to start with only one situation that you expect to encounter in the next week or so. Prepare a plan to handle it, applying what you have already learned about self-help. If necessary, review previous chapters for specific suggestions or ask your helpers for advice. If certain people are directly involved, you might want them to participate in planning and implementing the necessary changes. For example, if you are married and have children, the whole family could plan a vacation that would allow everyone to enjoy their favorite physical activities. Or if your roommate or spouse buys the groceries, sit down with them and decide how to reduce the calorie cost and food quantities they purchase for you.

After you've developed a thoughtful and realistic proposal, implement it for a week or so and see if it works. If it does, feel good about it. Pat yourself on the back and treat yourself extra nice. You deserve it! On the other hand, if you're still having trouble, you must keep up your commitment. Look at what happened, think it over, and prepare additional changes. Continue this process until the situation improves. Having come this far, you're bound to succeed.

Perhaps a case will illustrate the method. Sandy first pinpointed situations that were her weak areas. She selected drinking high-calorie beverages as her first problem because it occurred almost every day. After she developed a realistic plan, she implemented and evaluated it. Look at Table 10–2, "Situation 1," to see what she did.

Sandy also ate excessively at certain restaurants. She learned to control her intake at home but still had difficulty when eating out. Her solution and evaluation are recorded in Table 10–2. You can see by reviewing the table that she identified other problems too. We've left some of her proposed changes blank for you to think about. What would you recommend to Sandy?

TABLE 10-2
Overcoming Special Eating Situations: Sandy, A Case Illustration

Special Problem Situation	Proposed Changes	Evaluation
1. Drinking Beverages		
(a.) Too much coffee with cream and sugar.	(a.) Switch to artificial sweeteners and low fat milk. (See Chap. 5)	(a.) No problem. Coffee tastes about the same.
(b.) My spouse asks me to have before-dinner cocktails. I sometimes drink a cocktail even if I do not want one.	(b.) Keep more diet colas on hand and use instead. If I have a cocktail, I'll limit myself to one without sugary mixers. (See Chap. 8) I'll ask my spouse not to ask me to have a drink. (See Chap. 7)	(b.) Cut out more than half the cocktails I used to have. I felt good about asserting myself.
(c.) Sometimes I drink more alcohol than I need at parties.	(c.) Learn to "nurse" my drinks, to drink more slowly, and enjoy it more. (See Chap. 8.)	(c.) Found myself becoming more aware of how fast I used to drink. Had to tell myself to slow down last weekend. I did.
2. Eating Out		
(a.) Sunday brunches at the Pancake House have got to go.	(a.) We'll try that new coffee shop in town. See what it's like. (See Chaps. 7 and 8)	(a.) Food was only so-so. Not too many low calorie dishes either. We'll try another place next time.
(b.) It's hard to skip dessert when I know it's already paid for on the dinner	(b.) Tell myself the dessert is less important than meeting my weight goal. I'll try to eat slower too — not rush through dinner (See Chap. 8)	(b.) It wasn't easy but I said "no." I felt good about it too. Was my husband surprised!
3. Holidays and Vacations		
(a.) Stop all exercising (b.) Too many sweets and rich pastries around the house at Christmas and other special occasions.	(a.) Plan a vacation where there are opportunities for physical activity and rest. (See chap. 6)	
4. Skinny Friends or Spouse Are Always Eating		
(a.) This is a problem for me. My helpers have not been very supportive.		
5. The Rising Cost of Food		
(a.) Prepared diet foods are expensive		

Having served as Sandy's helper, now help yourself. Select one of your troublesome situations and write it down in Table 10-3, under "Special Problem Situations." Then think of concrete, realistic solutions and enter them in the column, "Proposed Changes." For at least the next week implement your plan and see if it doesn't help.

Don't go on to other situations until you've mastered the first one—and even then take them one at a time. If this lesson takes you several weeks to complete—depending on the number and types of problems you identify—*don't worry* ! In the long run the investment will be well worthwhile.

THE WEIGHT PLATEAU:
A TEMPORARY HOLDING AREA

Most people on diets want to see daily weight loss. When they step on the scale each day, they want it to read lower than the day before. When the reading is the same or higher, they sometimes feel frustrated and discouraged. Unfortunately, the reaction is often unwarranted. People very often lose weight steadily and then "plateau"—that is, not lose any weight for a week or more. Many factors cause a plateau effect.

1. weighing under different conditions,
2. greater water retention,
3. decreased physical activity, or
4. increased food intake.

Weighing under different conditions can cause your weight to fluctuate from one to six pounds. For example, last week you may have weighed yourself on Monday morning before breakfast, without any clothes on, after going to the bathroom. Two

TABLE 10–3

Overcoming Your Difficult Eating Situations

Special Problem Situations	*Proposed Changes*	*Evaluation*
1. Drinking non-alcoholic and alcoholic beverages		
2. Eating Out		
3. Holidays and Vacations		

TABLE 10-3
Overcoming Your Difficult Eating Situations

Special Problem Situations	Proposed Changes	Evaluation
4. Your skinny friends or spouse are always eating		
5. Dieting and the rising cost of food		
6. Others (specify)		

weeks later you may have weighed yourself Sunday evening after dinner, with your clothes on, and before going to the bathroom. Though at the end of two weeks you thought you weighed more, you may actually have lost two or three pounds of fat. But because the weigh-in conditions were completely different, you just didn't realize it. You may weigh yourself anytime you want, as long as the conditions are the same each time. Ideal times are just before going to bed in the evening or just after waking up in the morning.

Water temporarily retained by the body may show up as weight on the scale, even though your fatty tissue has been reduced. The water retention level can be affected by what you eat, particularly salty foods, which tend to increase water retention. If you weigh yourself in the morning after eating a heavily salted dinner and snack the previous evening, don't be surprised if you haven't lost weight. Try reducing your salt intake, and the plateau will disappear. Also, the one to five pounds women can gain during their menstrual period may hide actual fat loss. A loss of water weight will usually show up on subsequent weigh-ins, however. Diuretics should be taken only under a physician's supervision.

The breakdown of adipose tissue into useable energy is a complex conversion process that takes time. Some of the by-products are water molecules. If a lot of water is in your system, you may not lose any weight on the scale, when in fact your supply of fat is dwindling. The weight loss, however, will show up eventually if you expend more calories than you consume. Though not neccessarily consistent from week to week, it's bound to occur.

Plateau effects may also be due to unnoticed reductions in physical activity and/or to subtle increases in caloric intake. After being on a weight control program for a while, sometimes slipping back into old habits becomes easy, gradually eating more and exercising less without even being aware of it.

If you don't lose weight for a week or more, check to make sure your scale is accurate and that you weigh in consistently.

Reduce your salt intake and continue on your program for two more weeks. If you still aren't losing, you've probably let some old habits get the best of you. To avoid a tailspin, go back to your eating diary. Record everything you eat and every physical activity you do. Evaluate this information to see where slip-ups are occurring, and then take corrective action.

CONTINUE REWARDING YOURSELF AND GETTING HELP FROM YOUR FAMILY AND FRIENDS

Firmly establishing new eating, exercise, and life style habits, and finally reaching your weight goal will probably take a long time. For this reason, keep rewarding yourself along the way for each small change, for each new success. After all, you've worked hard and stuck to your commitment so far. You deserve a kind word. We also suggest that you continue to work with your helpers and to enlist support from family and friends; you can derive strength from them. Also remember to reward or thank your helpers for assisting you—they like to be appreciated just as you do.

If you've come this far, despite a setback here or there, you should be well on your way to living a brand new life, one in which you are both thinner and feel better about yourself. The last step now is to maintain your success, and the maintenance of the new you is the subject of the next chapter.

11

Maintaining The New You: Keeping It Off

By now you know that your *eating and activity patterns, not* your pounds, represent the real and continual problem. Hopefully either you are well on the way to reaching your weight goal, or you have reached it by now. This achievement has no doubt cost you a great deal of time, effort, and patience. So congratulations upon completing the previous chapters and, more important, upon eliminating at least some old fat habits and developing some new thin ones! You should feel very good about yourself. Will you celebrate by stopping your weight loss program because you no longer need to watch your weight?

No way!

In fact, your task is just beginning, though it should become easier and easier. To lose weight permanently—to keep it off for good—means to continue your new eating, exercise, and life style habits. You have done a great deal to take weight off, and the worst thing for you, physically and emotionally, would be *not* to keep it off. We will therefore review these new habits, present a remedial program if a relapse should occur (and it probably will), and discuss integrating the new you with the old you.

Once you reach your weight loss goal, you will have come the shortest and easiest lesson to perform in this book. You *stabilize* your weight by creating a balance between caloric intake and caloric expenditure. In effect, you may eat a *little* more than while you were losing weight. We recommend that you increase your caloric intake by about two to three hundred calories a day for a few weeks to see if your weight stabilizes.

If you want to be precise about this additional intake, increase your intake by one food calorie plan (see Chapter 5). If you are on a 1,200-calorie plan, go to a 1,500-calorie plan. If you are still losing weight, then move up to an 1,800-calorie food plan.

If you want to be more informal, simply add a *little* food to your regular intake and see what happens over a two- to four-week period. If you're still losing weight, add a little more. When you stop losing weight, *stop* adding food to your diet.

Notice that we have not recommended decreasing your physical activity as a way to stop losing weight. Though a possibility, physical activity is good for you in so many ways, besides losing weight, that we strongly urge you to continue as vigorous a physical activity program as is enjoyable.

PERMANENTLY ESTABLISHING YOUR NEW EATING, EXERCISE AND LIFE STYLE HABITS

Most people, when they reach their weight loss goal, tend to stop their diets and go back to their old habits. The reaction is quite understandable: After all, they've succeeded. But wait, have they really? If you go back to old habits, in a short time you'll also be back to your old weight. To prevent gaining weight again you must build permanent habit changes into your life. You do *not,* however, have to follow our suggestions rigidly; being flexible and open to trying things is crucial.

Basically use the same method you've used throughout the program. We have emphasized a general problem-solving approach by which you honestly assess your difficulties, set realistic goals, plan a reasonable program, try the program out for awhile, and evaluate what happened. You then modify your plans until the program works for you. To help you evaluate your overall progression and areas of continuing difficulty, review your status in regard to Chapters 4 through 10. These chapters comprise six basic content areas:

1. self-regulation;
2. taking in calories and diet management;
3. using up calories and physical activity;
4. getting support from family and friends; and
5. managing food; and
6. handling your feelings without eating.

You've probably completely mastered some of the principles in these chapters, while having occasional or continual problems with others. The "Progress Chart" in Table 11-1 will help you quickly assess your current successes. In column A put a " + " by each item you have mastered completely and a " – " by each item you have *not* mastered completely. Put a " + – " if you have difficulty with it sometimes. In column B write a summary comment of your status on that item.

Look over your progress chart carefully. You should feel good about all the pluses since they mean you've mastered these essential tasks of life-long weight control. You should feel good about yourself. Keep up the good work!

The items with plus/minuses or only minuses mean you

still have some work ahead. That's okay. Indeed they're expected since none of us are perfect. In this chapter you should *experiment* with new solutions to these problems until you have them under control.

As always, work on just one problem at a time. Propose a solution to it, try out the solution for about a week, then evaluate what happened. If you are successful, tell yourself, "I knew I could control it." Then reward yourself with something nice. If you don't succeed, re-evaluate the problem and propose another solution. With time and patience you'll eventually succeed.

Some of the activities in Chapters 4 through 10 may still be difficult to do regularly, such as handling your feelings of frustration and anger without eating. If you find yourself occasionally reverting to old habits, the best thing to do is to *repeat the relevant chapter and keep trying.* When you re-do the chapter, ask yourself what went wrong, and incorporate your thoughts into your second pass. Some chapters are harder than others. Go through the chapters *more slowly* this time. Repeat them as many times as necessary until you succeed. If you have to, reread and repeat things. We don't expect you to be perfect and you shouldn't either. Instead, congratulate yourself for trying again. You are all the time getting closer to permanent and healthy life style habits.

Let's take another case. Judy completed Chapters 4 through 9. She mastered a number of the tasks completely and felt proud of herself for doing so. Even though she had occasional problems refusing food at dinner parties, she soon learned to tell her hostess, "No thank you, I am on a diet and don't want any seconds or desserts." However, it was more difficult for her to say "No thank you" to her overweight next-door neighbor who frequently brought her freshly baked foods. She reread Chapter 7 on getting support from family and friends, and proposed a solution to this problem. The example in the "Trouble-Shooting Maintenance Record" (in Table 11–2) summarizes how Judy handled this touchy situation.

TABLE 11-1

Keeping-It-Off Progress Chart

	A. Check *"Plus"* *or* *"Minus"*	B. *Comments*

1. *Self-Regulation:* Do you self-observe, set realistic goals, and reward yourself?
 	
  a. Self-awareness observing
  b. Setting realistic goals
  c. Self-reward		

2. *Caloric Intake and Diets:* Do you control your caloric intake in a reasonable manner?
 	
  a. Common sense diet, or
  b. Food exchange diet		

3. *Physical Activity:* Do you expend or burn calories at home, at work, in traveling, and in recreation?
 	
  a. Home
  b. Work
  c. Traveling
  d. Recreation		

4. *Have you enlisted support from family and friends?*
 	
  a. Helper #1 _____
  b. Helper #2 _____
  c. Other _____
  d. _____		

	A. Check "Plus" or "Minus"	B. Comments
5. *Food Management:* Do you now buy, store, prepare, serve, eat, clean up, and snack low-calorie, high-nutrition, delicious food?		
a. Buying		
b. Storing		
c. Preparing		
d. Serving		
e. Eating		
f. Cleaning-up		
g. Snacking		
6. *Are you able to handle your feelings without eating?*		
a. Exhaustion		
b. Anxiety		
c. Boredom		
d. Loneliness		
e. Anger		

At this point you should write into the space provided in Table 11-2 all *your* problem behaviors and your proposed solutions to each of them. You've already pinpointed your problem areas by the minuses you checked on your "Keeping-It-Off Progress Chart" (Table 11-1). Now take *one* problem at a time and try to solve it. First take problem 1 and try your proposed solution for a week or more to see how it goes. *After* you have mastered this problem, go on to the next one and repeat the same process. If you do not solve it, then evaluate what happened, and propose another solution. Before reading further, continue this try-and-see approach until you have found a reasonable solution to each of your problem behaviors.

TABLE 11–2

Trouble-Shooting Maintenance Record

Problem Behavior	Proposed Solution	Evaluation
Example: *Judy-unable to say "no thanks" to neighbor who offers food.*	Example: *1. Have helper tell neighbor I am on diet and do not want her to offer me food.* *2. Tell neighbor this and thank her for cooperating.*	Example: *1. Neighbor at first upset but soon understood and no longer gives me fattening foods.* *2. I feel proud and rewarded myself by going to show with helper.*
Behavior 1:		
Behavior 2:		
Behavior 3:		
Behavior 4:		
Behavior 5:		

(If you need more writing space, insert blank sheets of paper)

IF YOU GAIN WEIGHT, DO
SOMETHING IMMEDIATELY

Contrary to popular beliefs, most normal-weight people must watch their weight regularly. If you talk with several such people, you will probably find that most of them continue to monitor their weight and take corrective action whenever they gain a few pounds above their normal weight. They usually watch their weight by weighing themselves regularly. Sometimes, they use the "pants test": Simply being aware of when their pants or skirts feel tight in the waist tells them that they have gained weight. This cue prompts them to go immediately on a corrective program. For example, they may eliminate desserts, reduce the quantity of food served, not take seconds, or order low-calorie meals at restaurants. They may also increase their physical activity. But they *do something immediately,* while losing one or two pounds is still easy.

How many times, after gaining a few pounds, were you unaware of it or dismissed it as only water retention or otherwise temporary? You weren't concerned, but before you knew it, you gained ten, maybe fifteen pounds. Perhaps you became so upset that you used your favorite way of handling stress—eating—and then gained another five or ten! Pretty soon you had gained fifteen to twenty-five pounds and were now desperate about losing weight.

Such instances point up the importance of awareness and self-observing in weight control (see Chapter 2). You must keep aware of your weight and take immediate action the day you gain weight. To assist you, we have provided a weekly weight graph in Appendix I. Cut it out along the dotted line and post it at a convenient, noticeable location such as on your refrigerator or clothes closet door. Write on the graph, where it says "weight," your maintenance weight. Then with a red pencil or marker draw a straight line across the graph *two* pounds above your maintenance weight. These two pounds represent your margin of safety; the red line, "Danger!" It tells you to look out for trouble may be ahead. Any weight above this line is dangerous to your long-term maintenance and should be treated immediately while the problem is still relatively easy.

Each week without fail, weigh yourself on the same day, at the same time, and in the same type of clothing. Record your weight on the graph for that week. After a few weigh-ins, you may see marginal fluctuations of a pound or two each week.

Alan's weekly weight graph is included to give you an idea of what a weekly record looks like (Figure 11–1). You can see that he maintained his weight with little variation for five weeks. Greater fluctuations happened the following five weeks, then in the eleventh week, he went four pounds over his maintenance weight. Rather than denying that he gained four

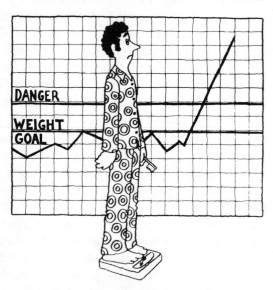

IF YOU GAIN WEIGHT, DO SOMETHING IMMEDIATELY

Courtesy of Dannon Milk Products. Used by permission.

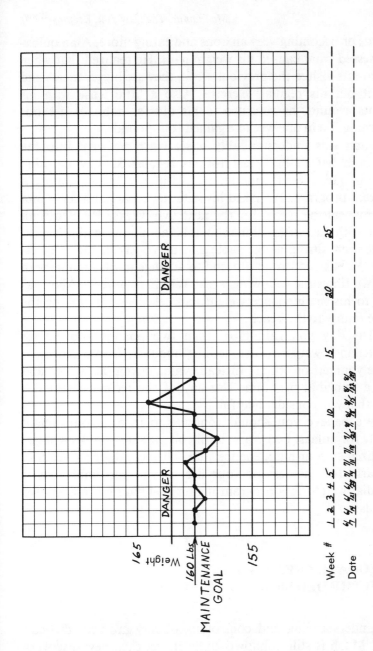

Alan's weekly weight graph.

199

pounds or becoming very anxious and eating more, Alan quickly assessed what caused his weight gain. He realized that when his parents visited the previous week, they ate bigger meals and he cut out his regular exercise. Also a little tense with his parents around, he returned to his old fat habit of nervous munching. So in one week he gained four pounds.

Alan was understandably upset when he went into the bathroom before breakfast for his regular Sunday morning weigh-in. He talked the matter over with his wife and planned a remedial program. He asked his wife to prepare and serve him only low-calorie meals for the next two weeks. He also took walks with her after dinner to talk about his parent's visit rather than sitting at the table and nervously eating the leftovers. He also called up a friend to arrange to play tennis with him two times the following week. Within two weeks Alan was back to his maintenance weight and celebrated by taking the whole family to the beach.

The day you gain more than two pounds above your maintenance weight, do something about it. Don't lament or blame yourself or others. Instead evaluate what happened and start a remedial program. Use any of the techniques in this book that you consider helpful.

We believe you should continue to record your weight weekly for at least two years, until you are sure your weight has stabilized at your maintenance goal. Then continue to weigh-in regularly for the rest of your life so you can implement a remedial weight loss program if ever you gain more than two pounds.

INTEGRATE THE NEW SELF WITH THE OLD SELF

Understanding and controlling obesity are very difficult tasks. Much is still unknown about it, yet each new discovery offers hope for a more effective treatment. Fortunately, enough is known to offer a realistic, scientifically based treatment program for losing weight and keeping it off. There is no easy way to lose weight. You must become involved, you must be commited and remain so, you must be willing to work to take it off and keep it off.

We have come a long way. We have presented a great deal of material and have asked you to make a great many changes in your life. The treatment program started by asking whether you were ready to lose weight, followed by a lesson on setting realistic goals and rewarding yourself for step-by-step success. You read a chapter on taking in calories and diets, and then one on using up calories and physical activity. You were given experience in understanding how other people affect your weight and how you can enlist their help. There was a chapter on how eating is the last link in a chain of actions leading up to excessive eating. You were presented with thin, less fattening ways to buy, store, prepare, serve, snack on, and clean up food. Understanding your feelings was highlighted—how they may lead to excessive eating and non-fattening ways to cope with your feelings. Also, attention was given to special eating situations and how you can handle them without having to overeat.

In short, we have asked you to become much more aware of what you do—your life-style—that contributes to your weight. We asked you to plan realistic programs for change, to implement your programs, to evaluate their effectiveness, and to make relevant alterations until the procedures work for you. You probably were already doing some of the activities we have asked you to do, others you might have done previously, and still others perhaps you had never done.

To lose weight permanently, many of these activities (but not all) must become *part of your daily life style.* With this accomplishment, you will be living a thinner, healthier, more vigorous life. You should feel excited, proud of your efforts—and reward yourself for your progress. You may already *think* of yourself as a thinner, leaner, healthier person. That's super—your mind is in tune with your body.

Sometimes, however, when persons change their overt behaviors, they don't immediately change their perceptions or attitudes about themselves. Often their thoughts, feelings, and self-images lag behind. For example, we have seen persons who have lost fifty to a hundred pounds, who look strikingly thinner and more attractive, yet who still perceive themselves as fat, ugly, and unattractive.

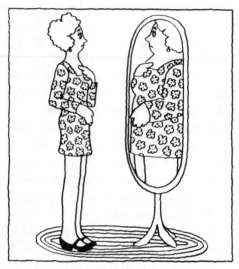

BRINGING YOUR BODY AND MIND TOGETHER

Courtesy of Dannon Milk Products. Used by permission.

You may experience this self-image lag also. Look at yourself. Do you emphasize the many successes you have accomplished? Do you feel proud of the changes you have made? Have you integrated these changes into your self-perceptions? Deception isn't helpful. Be honest with yourself: Yes or no? Do you emphasize the few failures you have encountered, feel ashamed of yourself, and still view yourself as fat and ugly? Yes or no? If you have already integrated your behavior changes and perceptions of yourself—great! Keep them together.

If you haven't yet integrated the two, they will need to be brought together. We know from research that *if you are to maintain all the outer behavioral changes, you must also make changes in the inner self as well.* The inner changes typically follow the behavioral changes, so give yourself some more time. Emphasize your accomplishments and reward them richly. You deserve something nice! Look back at Chapter 4 on setting realistic goals and rewarding successes. Review the positive realistic rewards for losing weight in Chapter 3, Table 3-1, and continue to emphasize all the benefits for staying thin. You are on the road to life-long maintenance.

Yet some people still feel worthless or unhappy, even after they have lost a great deal of weight and have received many of the positive benefits for being thinner. Though they think about their successful habit changes and the positive benefits of losing weight, they don't feel any better. This reaction sometimes indicates that other important things in a person's life have not been resolved by losing weight. Mary, for example, lost a great deal of weight and realized many of the benefits. She felt thinner and leaner . . . she could wear a smaller size dress . . . she received a great deal of social reinforcement from her friends for losing weight . . . she felt more attractive to the opposite sex . . . she appeared "normal" in appearance at her job. Yet, she still felt socially inadequate and fearful in interactions with men. Even though she was now more "sexy looking," she still had her same sexual hangups. Even though she was now thinner, she wasn't any less self-conscious at her job, any more socially competent, or promoted any faster at work.

Losing weight has many, many benefits, but it does not solve other problems in life. These problems still have to be faced and handled. If you have not lost weight, or have had difficulty keeping it off, we strongly recommend that you carefully re-examine your reasons for losing weight (Chapter 3, Table 3-1). Carefully review your positive realistic reasons for losing weight. Perhaps you will see some reasons that are now unrealistic. For example, even though you lose weight you probably will not have more friends or be promoted more readily at work.

After reviewing your reasons, you may discover that in addition to losing weight you may need to make some other changes in your life. Perhaps you want to have more friends. Maybe you'd like to be less anxious. Or your marriage or career might not be up to your expectations. Problems not related to weight loss are common. But you can make other changes in your life besides those in your eating and exercise habits. In fact, you can apply the same self-control approaches to these other concerns in your life.[1] Become aware of the factors contributing to your problem, set realistic goals, make plans for altering your physical and social environment as well as the environment inside yourself, and reward yourself for each small success.

In working through this book you may have realized that some personal problems are very difficult to solve by reading, doing tasks in a book, and talking with friends. That's all right; almost everybody has a period in his or her life that is difficult to cope with. If you have some of these personal concerns and would like to resolve them, then we encourage you to seek professional counseling. Consult your family physician, a psychologist, or a community mental health center for assistance.[2]

We hope the material so far has assisted you in looking at and helping yourself. As beautiful as life is, so is it short. You

---

[1] You may want to read some of the books listed in the references under self-management. These books also use a self-control approach to such problems as excessive drinking, fears, smoking, insomnia and other sleep problems, and female sexual problems.

[2] You can locate a psychologist by checking the classified section of the telephone directory or by calling a local mental health center for referral information.

deserve to give yourself now a thinner, healthier, happier, and possibly longer life. By applying the procedures described in this book you can take off and keep off those unwanted pounds. Losing weight and keeping it lost can be a powerful step in the direction of living a more satisfying life.

The next chapter discusses ways to apply our methods to two or more people. If you haven't already gone through it, you might benefit by doing so now.

12

Weight Loss For Two Or More

Traveling the road of permanent weight loss does not have to be lonely. Other people can join you. Dieting partnerships are an option you may want to explore with this program—and one that can have real benefits for you.

The current popularity of diet groups is reflected by Weight Watchers, TOPS (Take Off Pounds Sensibly), Overeaters Anonymous, Diet Watchers, and other commercial weight loss organizations. Each of them offers a congenial atmosphere, companionship, healthy competition, and a rich supply of useful suggestions for people who want to lose weight. Each of them also capitalizes on *mutual self-help*. More than any specific dietary plan, simply dieting with others is probably the main reason for their success and appeal.

Obviously, getting consistent attention and approval from others can understandably help in many ways. Although dieting with other people is not necessary for successful weight loss, it can increase your commitment and make a difficult task less burdensome. The friendly support of others is a powerful agent for change.

Although your helpers should be providing you with a source of support, helpers need not be skinny onlookers without a weight problem of their own. They too can be trying to lose weight, allowing you to be their helper just as they are yours. One of the best ways to learn how to lose weight permanently is to *teach* someone else how to do it.

SELECTING A WEIGHT LOSS PARTNER OR PARTNERS

If you feel your commitment needs a boost, or if you decide to look for a weight loss partner for other reasons, there are a few things to consider. First, your partner should be someone you like—a person you feel comfortable with and can talk with freely. Trying to diet, let alone talk about heaviness with some people, may give rise to defensive behavior, hurt feelings, and misunderstanding. If you think certain of your friends could present such problems, you are probably better off looking for a partner elsewhere.

Another consideration is access and availability. The person you select should be one you see frequently (at least once or twice a week) at home, at work, or in the neighborhood. Partnerships apart have a way of becoming no partnership at all. Opportunities for regular interaction should be made available.

A third and final consideration is the motivation of your partner—to either lose weight or to stick to some other mutually negotiated arrangement. Without dedication, an initial burst of enthusiasm ("Let's do it!") can turn quickly to indifference and eventually lead to a breakdown in your arrangements.

Because a parting of the ways can disrupt your plans—and lower your commitment too (dropping out can be contagious)—avoid too quick an arrangement.

Maybe you have more than one person with whom you would like to form a partnership. For example, perhaps several friends in the neighborhood or at work have talked about losing weight and are also willing to do something about it. Similarly, other members of the family may want to join the program you have started, especially if you have started to set a good example.

Weight loss partnerships can involve more than two people. Groups should be small enough to manage, so they can meet regularly and provide an overall sense of companionship, as well as allow for personal involvement: You don't want people to feel lost in the crowd. But beyond that requirement no specific rules govern group size. In fact groups larger than two people have the advantage of offering more positive support and a variety of favorable models too.

Table 12–1 is for you to use in selecting potential weight loss partners. Write down the names of a few people who might be interested in pursuing a dietary program with you. For each name you put down, ask yourself, "Can I work with that person?" In doing so, keep in mind the considerations discussed above.

You should also remember that "instant" partners are usually available by joining a commercial diet group such as Weight Watchers. While these groups can be helpful,[1] they are also somewhat expensive (about $150 a year in Weight Watchers) and you can't tell who your partners will be. What about your spouse, your teenage son or daughter, your neighbor or friend? Any one of them could turn out to be a good partner for you.

---

[1]Evaluative information regarding the success of at least one self-help group (TOPS) has been reported by Levitz and Stunkard. The complete reference is in the back of this book.

TABLE 12-1
My List of Potential Partners

Name	Can I Work Well with Person?
1.	
2.	
3.	
4.	
5.	

CONTRACTING FOR CHANGE

Once you've selected a partner, you're ready to take some action *together*. But what should the two (or more) of you do? Basically *stick with the general program in this book. Whether you're dieting alone or with others makes no difference, because in either case you must concentrate on changing your eating and exercise habits before you can expect permanent weight loss.* This emphasis on habit change must always be kept in mind, as well as the fact that these changes take time.

Dieting with other people, however, does present a different situation and therefore calls for new techniques. Our method for dealing with diet partnerships is called a *behavioral contract,* or simply *contracting for change.*

WHAT'S A CONTRACT?

According to Webster's dictionary, a contract is "an agreement between two or more people for doing or not doing something specified." In other words, a contract describes *who will do what for whom under what conditions.*

Most contracts, by definition, involve an exchange between people "of something for something." For example, when you borrow money from the bank to purchase a car, you enter a contract with the representatives of the bank. By that contract, the bank officials agree to let you use some of the bank's money in return for your guaranteeing them repayment of the money itself plus a "usage charge"—the interest. If you don't live up to the contract, the car may be repossessed. Similarly, when you visit doctors or dentists, they agree to provide certain services in exchange for a fee. Although less formal than a bank contract, the arrangement is still a contract.

Implicit contracts also occur between family members, friends, and the like. They are often unstated, almost never formalized in writing, and in fact usually evolve through trial and error. But just like other (legal) contracts they influence what we do. Many married couples, for example, have an implicit understanding of what they will do if one is going to be late getting home: The late arriving spouse will call the other so he or she won't worry and become angry. Likewise, a teenager who borrows the family car knows that he must be home by midnight if that privilege is to continue. Both of these examples are implicit contracts: The expected behaviors and consequences are informally understood.

Although contracts often involve an exchange of positive things (privileges, favors, services), they can also be *coercive* in nature. One or both parties may use threats or punishment to influence the behavior of the other. The ultimatum is, "You better do it or something bad is going to happen." Examples of implicit coercive contracts include, "Keep the house clean or

I'll tell you what a terrible homemaker you are . . . Show me affection *now* or I won't talk to you for a week . . . Hurt me and I'll hurt you back . . . Lose weight or I'll keep on nagging you.'' In each case one person is coerced into doing or not doing something by fear or threats of punishment from the other—all negative consequences.

Although commonly used to motivate others, coercive contracts are not nearly as effective as *positive contracts,* because one person is forced to do something. Eventually the ''loser'' may decide to fight back (''I'm not going to do it . . . Why don't you get off my back?'') or leave the relationship altogether. Hence the contract breaks down. At that point the other party loses too. A much more satisfactory arrangement occurs when both parties *want* to do something because nice things happen when they do.

BEHAVIORAL CONTRACTS: A TOOL FOR CHANGE

Contracts can be used to resolve existing conflicts or to further the attainment of specific wants and goals.[2] To illustrate, let's consider a recent case described by Peter Miller, a behavioral psychologist. In this instance a husband and wife found themselves in a constant battle over his excessive drinking after he returned home from work in the evening. He would drink, and she would nag—which the husband detested to no end. Unfortunately the strategy did not work; neither person was willing to change. After the ritual had continued for some time, threatening the very existence of the marriage, the husband and wife finally decided to seek professional help. Miller suggested that a *behavioral contract* be drawn up between them, one mutually negotiated so that it was satisfying to both persons. After some further discussion, and a little ''give and

[2]For additional information on behavioral contracts you might want to consult the book by DeRisi and Butz in the reference section.

take,'' the husband agreed to limit his drinking to an amount acceptable to his wife; she didn't necessarily want a teetotaler but felt that three drinks was enough for one evening. In return she would refrain from her nagging.

To keep both parties honest, they also agreed that a penalty would be imposed for failure to live up to their bargain. Thus the husband agreed to forfeit twenty dollars each time he exceeded his drinking limit, which his wife could spend in as frivolous a way as possible; she agreed to pay the same penalty to her husband if she nagged. (The couple had separate checking accounts.) The arrangement was formalized in writing and signed by both parties. In this way there was never any accusation of "That's no fair—I never realized that." Within a short time, in fact a matter of days, both husband and wife had changed their ways in a manner that was *mutually* satisfying and consistent with their individual wants.

Similar contractual arrangements have been used to motivate other kinds of behavior change: better cooperation between parents and their children, helping smokers break the cigarette habit, increasing academic performance in students, even treating drug abusers. And, of course, behavioral contracts have also been used to facilitate weight loss in overweight people.

WRITING A BEHAVIORAL CONTRACT

Writing a behavioral contract is not something to be done haphazardly or at a moment's notice. If it is, the contract is likely to fail. Instead, preparing a contract requires a lot of careful thinking and is best done in a step-by-step fashion. Essentially there are four steps involved.

1. First, *bring together two or more people* who are interested in changing their respective behavior and in helping

each other in the process. As you'll see, the type of change desired may be the same or different for each person.

2. The second step, *negotiating goals,* is probably the most important as well as the most difficult. Carefully specify what each person wants from the contract, and what they will be expected to do to get it. Thoughtful discussion, sharing of ideas, an attitude of fairness, and above all, mutual compromise are needed to accomplish this talk.

3. The third step involves the identification of a set of *consequences* for compliance *and* noncompliance with the contract. Compliance should result in something nice, a reward of some sort. On the other hand, failure to comply with the contract can be followed by a penalty or fine.

4. Finally, *formalize the agreement* by putting it in writing and having each party sign the written document. To insure that each party remembers the terms of the contract, copies can be made available to each participant.

Some of you may find the idea of a written contract objectionable. Perhaps the idea seems to mechanical, too artificial, even childlike. If you feel this way, you might prefer to use an oral agreement or to work with your partner using no contract at all. Either of these methods is fine. Whether they *work* for you and your partner is the important consideration. You might want to try an arrangement other than a written contract first and see how it goes. Depending on the outcome, you can always switch to a written contract later on. Being flexible is perfectly acceptable, as long as it helps you get what you're after.

In the case of the married couple described earlier, step 2 consisted of the husband's limiting his drinking to three drinks nightly—a substantial reduction from his usual six to nine drinks before the contract was adopted. In exchange the wife agreed to refrain from nagging. The rewarding consequence, step 3, was the reciprocal change each desired in the other. However to prevent one party from reneging and to make it worthwhile for the other to stick to the bargain, a twenty-dollar fine was included as a consequence for noncompliance. Thus if the husband failed in his agreement, there would still be an *independent* consequence for his wife not to do the same. If she did, she would lose twenty dollars too.

As regards weight loss, a similar contract, for example, might read as follows:

> Husband agrees to reduce his daily caloric intake (as described in Chapter 5) so he can lose one pound per week, in exchange for his wife doing the same [we'll assume they *both* have an interest in losing weight and want to see their partner slimmer too]. Each week the husband meets his goals, his wife agrees to do something special (rewarding) for him; and conversely, when the wife meets her goals, he agrees to do something special for her. They both make a list of mutually agreed on nice things or pleasant activities which they will give to the other as rewards. If the husband fails to meet his goal, he helps his wife with the dishes each night of the following week. Conversely, if the wife fails, she mows the lawn and washes the cars [chores that were ordinarily her husband's responsibility].

NEGOTIATING A WORKABLE CONTRACT: TEN RULES

Behavioral contracts are an effective means of motivating behavior, but they have other advantages as well. For one, contracting teaches people that mutual changes in each other's behavior are negotiable, that things can get better. Because contractual goals are specified clearly in advance, they help the participants become more aware of their mutual responsibilities and the consequences of meeting or shirking those responsibilities. When expectations are clear-cut, many misunderstandings can be avoided. Above all, contracting encourages people to use an exchange of rewards, instead of threats, as a way of bringing desired changes about: Such a positive approach in itself can make life much more pleasant.

However, writing a fair and effective contract is no easy matter. Thoughtful negotiation takes time. If you have never written a contract before (and chances are you haven't), you might want to follow some rules of contracting.[3] They can make the task easier and the outcome more to your liking.

Rule 1. The contract payoff (reward) should be immediate.

Rule 2. Initial contracts should reward small approximations.

We've already talked about the problem of setting habit change and weight loss goals too high. Make sure the ones you set are realistic and within reach. Instead of writing a contract aimed only at achieving your long-term weight goal, write in clauses aimed also at achieving your short-term goals. From a learning standpoint, waiting too long for anything is neither helpful nor very much fun.

Rule 3. Reward frequently with small amounts.

Rule 4. The contract should reward accomplishment rather than obedience.

This distinction is essentially a value judgement, with the purpose of fostering self-reliance on the parties to the contract. Commanding "Do what I tell you" usually meets with obedience or disobedience, but the statement "If you accomplish such and such, *you* will earn . . ." generally encourages ac-

---

[3]These particular rules were adopted from a book about contracting written by Homme et al. (1969).

complishment. Of the two, the accomplishment is the preferable approach.

Rule 5. Reward performance after it occurs.

Rewards should not be given until after the desired behavior takes place or after goals are reached.

Rule 6. The contract must be fair.

The terms of the contract should be about *equal* for *all* parties involved. Furthermore, the amount of reward should be related to the amount of behavior requested or performed. A wife who insists that her husband take over all household duties for each week in which she changes her habits and loses one pound is not being fair. Conversely, a husband who insists that his wife lose twenty pounds before he will do any household chores isn't being fair either. The terms of the contract need to be negotiated in a way that each party believes the contract to be fair.

Rule 7. The terms of the contract must be clear.

Each party should know *exactly* what is expected of him or her, and what will happen as a result of compliance. As a check, having another person not involved in the contract read it over sometimes helps. If others cannot understand the terms of the arrangement, the contract probably needs to be made clearer.

Rule 8. The contract must be honest.

No cheating or welshing is allowed after an agreement is made.

Rule 9. The contract must be positive.

Benefits, gains, and rewards should be emphasized, while penalties or fines should be minimized.

Rule 10. Contracting as a method of change must be used systematically.

The term "systematic" means methodical, according to plan, consistent. If contracting becomes an on-again/off-again thing, it probably won't get you or your partner very far. Nor can a contract be systematic if you enter it without a sense of commitment or with at least the intention of trying hard to stick to the bargain you've made. This does not mean contracts cannot be renegotiated after they're begun, however renegotiation should only take place after some agreed upon time, not in midstream.

SOME EXAMPLES OF BEHAVIORAL CONTRACTS FOR WEIGHT MANAGEMENT

EXCHANGE OF SMALL GIFTS OR FAVORS

One method of contracting involves the exchange of small gifts, money, or special favors between partners for meeting their respective contract goals. The purposes of the contract are to specify goals and to enhance motivation by providing mutual support among the participants and by exchanging rewards after contract goals are met.

In a successful contract only winners emerge and no one comes out a loser. The goal is not for one partner to outdo the other, but for both partners to reach the goals they've set. Here's how this type of contract is established, step by step:

Step 1. Both partners determine their initial weight by weighing in with the other partner, so that things are kept on the up-and-up. They then record both amounts on the contract form.

Step 2.   Both partners agree to change some specific eating and exercise habits as well as to lose a specified amount of weight. Which habits to change or how much weight loss is desired is entirely a matter of individual choice. Chapters 4 through 9 provide suggestions on eating, exercise, and life style habits that are helpful to change.

In accordance with rule 2 (initial contracts should reward small approximations), set realistic, *weekly* goals, which then allow for weekly rewards if the goals are met. Also a completion or deadline date may be included for completing the long-term goals or for re-negotiating the contract. Once goals and deadlines are established, they are written into the contract.

Step 3.   Both partners agree to exchange a small gift or favor (of roughly equal value) immediately after their respective goals are met. (Look over Table 12–2 for a list of possible rewards.) If both partners meet their goals, they both win and the exchange takes place. However, if only one partner meets his goal, he alone is the winner. He receives his reward but he is not bound to give one in return. The nature of the rewards, or their approximate monetary value (for example, a gift costing no less than $5 and no more than $10) should also be specified in the contract.

Step 4.   After each partner fills in his or her own contract, and both partners agree to the terms of their participation, they sign the contracts. Copies of the contracts may then go to each partner.

An example of a general purpose behavioral contract for weight management is shown in Table 12–3. The details of the contract have been filled in by the two partners, Mary Smith and Susan Williams. Mary has set as her short-term *weekly* goals to lose one half to two pounds, to observe her caloric intake daily, to take in 1,200 or less calories per day on the average, to exercise weekly, and to work at changing specific eating habits. Weekly rewards for Mary include paying herself ten dollars,

TABLE 12-2

Some Possible Rewards for Meeting Contract Goals

money
going to a movie or a play
going to the beach
spending "extra" time at a favorite hobby
buying a favorite record album
playing certain sports
getting to be "boss" with the partner
spending extra time with a friend
reading or buying a desired book
going to a party
goofing off time
watching certain TV programs, or not watching them
getting a massage from partner
going out on the town (certain restaurant, show, dance spot, etc.)
making a special purchase (clothes, tools, an appliance)
taking lessons in something (music, crafts, sports, etc.)
going on a picnic (where, when, with whom)
variety in sexual behavior
box of stationery
bouquet of fresh flowers
going to a museum
going to a concert
going skiing
going on a trip somewhere
night out with the boys or girls
buying a poster or painting
getting to sleep in late
making something for partner
obtaining or caring for pets
receiving some other special favor from partner

(Use the space below to list some other rewards that you can think of)

1.

2.

3.

4.

5.

6.

7.

8.

9.

10.

TABLE 12-3

Behavioral Contract for Weight Management

This agreement, made and entered into this _14_ day of _Sept._, 19_77_, by and between _Mary Smith_ and _Susan William_.

Witnesseth:

A. *My Weight Management Goals:*

I, _Mary Smith_, have reviewed various possible weight management goals and have agreed to work hard at achieving the following, realistic goals. (Check off and fill in the details of only the goals that will be helpful to *you*.)

1. I will seek to lose between _½_ and _2_ pounds per week and continue to lose weight until I reach my weight goal of____pounds.

2. I will observe regularly my
   a. caloric intake   Yes _✓_   No____
   b. caloric expenditure   Yes _✓_   No____
   c. weekly weight   Yes _✓_   No____

3. I will keep my caloric intake, on the average, at _1200_ calories or less.

4. I will increase my weekly physical activities
   a. To use up _1000_ or more calories per week
   b. To do one or more of the following activities
      (1) _walking_   (3) _playing tennis_
      (2) _gardening_   (4) _biking_

5. I agree to work on the following eating habits
   a. _buy low calorie foods_
   b. _eat more slowly_
   c._____

6. I also agree to work on the following habit changes: (fill in any additional goals you want to achieve)
   a._____
   b._____
   c._____

B. *My Rewards and Consequences*

(Check off and fill in the details of only the consequences that will be helpful to *you*.)

1. I, *Mary Smith*, agree to make a total deposit of $*150*. I further agree to pay myself $ *10* of the total deposit each week I achieve my habit improvement and weight loss goals. If I do not make my weight improvement goals, I agree *not* to pay myself that week. Any money not earned back by the end of the program will be given to *United Way*.

2. I will reward myself weekly with one or more of the following activities. (List rewarding activities.)
   a. *take a hot bath*
   b. *go clothes shopping*
   c. *go to a movie*
   d._____
   e._____

3. My weight management partner, *Susan Williams*, agrees to do the following when I make my weekly goals.
   a. Praise me for my efforts *each week*.
   b. Do the following for me *(1) play tennis with me (2) babysit for my children so I can go out to the museum.*

4. When I do *not* make my weekly goals I agree to do the following:
   _____
   _____

5. Additional Consequences: _____
   _____

We have both read the above contract and agree to the goals and consequences checked. We both agree to follow the contract until the goals or review date are reached, whichever comes first. We may at that time renegotiate the contract.

First Partner: *Mary Smith*   Second Partner: *Susan Williams*

Current Date: *September 14, 197-*

Review Date: *December 14, 197-*

treating herself to a hot bath, going clothes shopping or to a movie, and telling herself that she has done a good job. Her weight partner, Susan, agrees to praise her for her efforts and play tennis with her, or babysit for Mary's children so Mary can go out to the museum. Note that some of the goals or consequences in the general purpose contract were not relevant to Mary, so she didn't include them in her contract. Susan filled in a similar contract and they both signed them. Appendix J contains several blank contracts for your use. If you want additional copies, cut one out along the dotted line and duplicate.

Before concluding this section, the issue of contract goals should be clarified. Seemingly weight loss and the maintenance of one's weight, is the most important goal to set; this is not necessarily so. While either goal is certainly relevant, the establishment of specific *habit change* goals are more important. For example, in your contract you should include realistic goals to increase your exercise a certain amount per week (as described in Chapter 6). Similarly, you should include goals to slow down your eating, to cut out certain snack breaks, or to reduce your intake of tempting but high-calorie foods. You might also want to contract for maintaining a lowered calorie intake according to the guidelines spelled out in Chapter 5. The important thing is to establish specific and realistic eating, exercise, and life style goals that help you lose weight and keep it off.

A TWO-DIMENSIONAL CONTRACT: WEIGHT LOSS AND HOUSEHOLD DUTIES[4]

A variation of the behavioral contract is the two-dimensional contract. The term "two-dimensional" refers to the contract's dual purpose: in this case to encourage weight

[4]This contractual arrangement was first proposed by Lutzker and Lutzker (1974). Our appreciation is extended for allowing us to borrow their ideas.

loss as well as the performance of household chores. Because this type of contract is intended for people who share household duties, it is most appropriate for married couples, a parent and child (such as a mother and her teenage daughter), roommates, or other pairings. Furthermore this contract is good to use when only one member of the partnership wants to lose weight. Under these conditions, however, the other partner must also value that goal and support bringing it about.

Essentially, a two-dimensional contract involves a temporary "vacation" from necessary but unpleasant household duties as a reward for meeting a weight loss or a habit change goal. As long as the dieter's goals are met, he or she gets to avoid doing unpleasant work. The reward for the other partner is a slimmer mate, plus the satisfaction of helping out. If the contract goals are not reached, the dieter's work load increases—the penalty for noncompliance.

How does a two-dimensional contract work? The first step is to make a complete list of routine household duties (for example, making the bed, clearing the dinner table, feeding the pets,taking out the trash, cleaning the bathroom, and so on). From this list each partner is assigned a set of chores, an agreed-upon division of labor. Delegation of responsibilities should be fair and may rotate from week to week so both partners have an equal share. Obviously, chores must still get done.

After chores are delegated, the partner who wants to lose weight or change eating habits weighs in to establish a starting weight. Then weekly habit change and weight loss goals are set. (One to two pounds a week is plenty.) All this information is then recorded in the contract.

The final step is negotiating consequences for reaching your goals as well as for not reaching your goals. In a two-dimensional contract, these consequences are selected from the list of household chores and exchanged according to the dieter's success or failure. For weight loss and successful habit change, the dieter might earn a week-long vacation from two chores of his or her choosing—washing the morning dishes, for example, and emptying the trash. On the other hand, if the terms of the contract are not met—such as no loss of weight or improvement of habits—the dieter agrees to take on additional chores of the *partner's choosing* for one week. After consequences are specified, they are written into the contract.

Two additional points need to be addressed. First, weight maintenance may be the goal of the contract, in which case it too should be rewarded, especially if relapses or weight gains have been a problem. Second, two-dimensional contracts are made to be renegotiated on a regular basis. At renegotiating time, weight goals, habit change goals, and/or consequences for goal attainment can be altered depending upon past progress, issues of fairness, or general need for further change.

If you want to try a two-dimensional contract, discuss it with your partner. If your partner agrees, fill in the relevant details in the blank contract in Appendix J and begin.

CONTRACTING FOR WEIGHT LOSS IN GROUPS

If you have more than one weight loss partner, the contracts discussed so far may be difficult to implement. Deciding who will do what for whom under what conditions can be a complicated matter for two people, let alone for more. However, other contracts can be used with threesomes or other small groups. Like other forms of contracting, the basic requirement for group agreements is the careful setting of goals and consequences.

Another requirement is that members attend scheduled group meetings, especially where weigh-ins and consequences occur. Obviously, group meetings can serve other useful purposes too. They may be an occasion for celebrating successful weight loss *together with the habit changes that produced it,* or they may be used to provide continued support and encouragement for others who are finding the tasks more difficult. Group meetings can also be an occasion to share interesting low-calorie recipes, to plan exercise outings, or just to have fun. However, only when weight loss partners attend meetings regularly will a sense of purpose and group spirit be developed and maintained.

A powerful reward for weight loss behavior is *money*. Just about everyone will work to obtain it or to avoid losing it. In a group setting, earning back money *that partners have deposited previously* is a rewarding consequence *par excellence*. For all practical purposes, the terms of the contract can be arranged so that people are literally paid for reaching the goals they've set.

Here's the way a contract for groups might work. The first step is forming a group and deciding where and how often it will meet: meetings once or, perhaps twice a week in the beginning are important. Whether the membership consists of husbands, housewives, singles, or sons and daughters makes little difference as long as group members are *commited to work together*.

Once a group is formed, the next step is for each person to establish short-term and long-range weight goals: the weight loss desired, the habit changes needed, and pace to set. The main concern is that weight goals should be tailored to individual needs and set at a level where they can be reached. (You might want to refer to Chapter 4 for a more complete discussion of realistic goal-setting.) Thus one person may want to lose a total of ten pounds at a rate of one pound a week, while increasing his or her exercise by participating more regularly in certain sports or activities. Both of these goals can be easily written into the contract. Similarly, another person may want to lose thirty pounds at two pounds a week, at the same time reducing troublesome eating habits such as between-meal snacking. A third person may want just to maintain his or her present weight but feel the need for some help in doing so. A contract is one way for all these persons to obtain help.

After goals are established, they should be recorded by a person who is appointed or elected by the group to be the group's *bookkeeper.* He or she records all contract goals, keeps track of the progress of group members toward those goals, and records all other official business (such as monetary transactions).

A motivating force behind the contract is money, a sum of which is deposited by each and every group member immediately after goals are set. The amount deposited will vary from person to person, but the amount should be large enough that the individual will want to recover it and will work to avoid losing it permanently. All deposits are recorded by the groups's bookkeeper as soon as they are collected; refunds, as weight loss occurs. The deposits can be used to open a checking account at a nearby bank, thus ensuring safekeeping of the money and also providing a convenient vehicle of earning it back gradually over a series of weeks.

Although money is a powerful and natural motivating consequence, it may not be appropriate in each and every case. For example, some people may not be able to afford a large outlay of cash, such as the unemployed teenager. Others may simply object to tying personal changes to dollars and cents. If any such circumstances arise, the watch-word is always *flexibility.* Non-money alternatives can also be used as rewarding consequences, as we've already indicated in this chapter. One example would be for group members to agree to do nice things or special favors for each other when weight goals are attained. Or perhaps a group member could substitute a certain amount of time in lieu of money; thus he or she might make a "deposit" of so many work hours (to help out on a project, to assist a charitable organization, maybe even to babysit) that could be earned or forfeited depending on the progress made. Though money is an incentive for most of us, it's certainly not the only one.

The final step in the contract follows logically from the others. Group members earn back their money or other agreed-upon rewards by meeting the goals they've set—by fulfilling the terms of the contract. If money is the reward, the rate at which it is earned back (such as ten percent installments over ten meetings or twenty percent over five meetings) depends on individual preference and the amount of weight loss desired. If someone's goal is to lose twenty-five pounds in two weeks, to expect that person to earn back his or her deposit in such a short period would be unreasonable and unhealthy. Spreading refunds out over a longer period for a series of small habit change and weight loss goals is the preferable route to take.

In order to make contracts binding, everyone should clearly understand that when contract goals are not met on schedule, the money to be earned is lost for that week. The entire deposit is not forfeited, only the money scheduled to be refunded for meeting a specific contract goal. At the end of the program, a person still has the option to earn back the unrefunded money if he or she has met the final habit change and weight loss goals. The contract should specify what will happen to any money not earned back.

Furthermore, and consistent with our emphasis on learning better *self-control*, each member of the group should be *personally responsible* for determining whether goals have been met and rewards earned at the end of a given week. If there is any room for doubt, the decision can always be made with the *assistance* of others, but the final decision rests with the individual. This approach teaches people to set realistic goals and to use rewards selectively, when they have been properly earned. It also reduces the chances of persons' becoming angry with the group, since each person has the final decision-making responsibility.

For example, Jennifer contracts with the group to play tennis with another group member once a week and to lose one or more pounds a week. If she reaches her goal she could earn back five dollars of her initial fifty-dollar deposit. However, if she fails to reach her goal on time, Jennifer should *not* reward herself; she loses the five dollars. Jennifer can still earn back the other forty-five dollars assuming future weekly contract goals are met, but she pays a price for noncompliance. This arrangement may sound overly harsh, but in the long run Jennifer learns that she must work harder to lose what she wants—more weight and less money!

Money lost for not meeting contractual goals can be put to good use. For example, it might go into a winner's pool and be used as a bonus reward for those who have accomplished their goals. The dividends could be split evenly or awarded in a lottery for which only winners are eligible. On the other hand, the money might finance a party, a special outing, or a contribution to a charitable organization. Regardless of how nonrefunded money is spent, the decision should be made jointly by all group members.

Of course, the uppermost goal of the group is for each person to bring about desired changes in themselves, *not* for some to profit at the expense of others. This point needs to be kept in mind constantly.

SUMMARY

We've talked about weight loss partnerships and how to increase your commitment to lose weight by dieting with others. The principal method we discussed was the behavioral contract, which involves mutual specification of goals (whether weight loss or habit changes) and an exchange *of* something *for* something. We described several different contract strategies, ranging from an exchange of small gifts or favors between two people to the use of monetary contracts in groups. Above all, contracting should be carried out with an attitude of fairness, compromise, and mutual self-help. When used in this way, contracting is a useful tool that many have found to be helpful. However, it's *not* a tool that everyone *must* use.

13

Improving Your Child's Eating Habits: Prevention At Its Best

Thus far we've considered weight problems in adults. For those of you who are parents, however, an equally important concern may be the weight of your children. In today's affluent, overindulgent society, few children are underfed. Except for those who live in severe poverty, most American children do not face the constant threat of starvation and malnutrition as children do in other countries. Instead, more and more children are overfed and overweight; some estimates put the number of overweight children in this country as high as thirty percent. They range from the chubby youngster who is just a few pounds too heavy to the rotund child who is obviously obese—perhaps more than fifty percent above the normal weight for his height and age. In the words of one pediatrician,[1] "Our society is becoming fatter earlier."

[1] See Eden (1975).

SOME FACTS ABOUT CHILDHOOD
OBESITY

Most fat children grow up to be fat adults. The earlier they become obese and the longer they remain overweight as youngsters, the more difficulty they have in losing weight later on. Only recently have some of the reasons for this effect become known: Without doubt, the most important factors are *poor eating habits* and *inadequate physical activity*. The so-called "glandular" hypothesis has been shown to be invalid for over ninety percent of obese children and adolescents. The biggest problem is the same as with adults: eating inappropriate foods too much and too often.

TOO MANY FAT CELLS?

One hypothesis currently under study is that when too many fat cells develop early in life, they never can be eliminated. Some researchers[2] believe that children who overeat develop a large number of fat cells in their body, certainly many more than their thinner peers. By seven years of age some obese youngsters may have already accumulated more fat cells in their bodies than full-grown, normal-weight adults. Of course, fat cells increase when we eat more than our bodies need is not surprising; what is surprising is that once these cells are formed early in life, they may be difficult to get rid of later on. The *hyper-cellularity* (or "too-many-fat-cells") hypothesis suggests that, while stringent dieting or normal growth spurts will produce weight loss, the reason is usually that the cells only shrink in size as their fat content is depleted. The fat cells themselves stay with the child, as if they were waiting to be filled up again.

[2]Recall the results of Hirsh, *et al.* in Chapter 1.

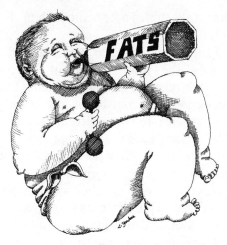

A fat baby may become a fat adult. Courtesy Smithsonian, *April, 1975.*

The implications of this theory are significant. One implication runs contrary to popular notions that a fat baby is a healthy baby or that overweight children *usually* grow out of their fat. By clinging to such beliefs, parents may be doing their children a grave disservice in the long run. Beware, however, against using the too-many-fat-cells hypothesis as an excuse or rationalization.

HOW CHILDREN LEARN TO BE OVERWEIGHT

Although obese children are often the product of overweight parents, this does *not* necessarily mean that their weight problems are inherited (that is, transmitted through the genes) nor that they are doomed to be fat because their parents were. Some overweight children have normal-weight parents, and some overweight parents have normal-weight children. Even among identical twins reared apart, one may become fat

232 *Improving Your Child's Eating Habits*

while the other stays thin. Factors other than the genes are obviously at work.

Family habit patterns of overeating and inactivity are probably among the most important factors. These are transmitted to children, not through the genes but through learning and experience. Children begin to learn about food very early in life. They learn to value certain foods and prefer them to others. They observe how and what their parents eat and may try to imitate them. They learn which foods taste good, look good, are in fact good for them. They even learn which foods have special symbolic significance, which contain prizes, or which can be used to purchase toys. In short, children learn a lot about what, when, and how much to eat by direct experience with the people and events around them.

Children also learn about the fun and enjoyment of regular exercise, such as how to play active sports, games, and hobbies. Conversely, some children learn that watching TV is the best way to spend their idle time. Most parents don't try to teach any of these lessons consciously; on the contrary, much learning occurs in spite of conscious intent. Recall the old saying, "Do as I say, not as I do." Well, the *doing* is what counts, though the process may be entirely accidental, taking place over a period of months or years. Unfortunately, the eating and activity habits that emerge are not always good. They may even be the same ones that you have been struggling to change. You might be wondering how this learning takes place in children. Table 13–1 provides some specific examples that usually lead to trouble later on.

WHAT PARENTS LEARN

Learning is not a one-way process. Parents learn something too. For example, if candy or snacks help to calm a child down, or they bring a smile to his face where tears were before, most parents will find these consequences highly rein-

TABLE 13-1
How Children Learn to Overeat

1. Millions of dollars are spent annually on television, newspapers, and magazine advertisements to tempt and encourage children to eat high-calorie food.

2. Access to fattening foods is made easy by buying them and keeping them around the house.

3. Too many junk foods are given as snacks. They soon become expected and preferred over more nutritious foods.

4. Too much time is spent in sedentary activities such as TV viewing. Too little positive instruction and encouragement is given for active play, regular exercise, and family sports.

5. Children are admonished to eat every bite. They are told to hurry up and eat, because others are waiting or the food will get cold. They are sometimes led to believe that if they don't clean their plates, they will hurt their parents' feelings or not grow big and strong. On top of this, more than one child has been made to feel guilty for *not* eating by moralistic spiels about the starvation that abounds in other countries.

6. Food is used to tranquilize children when they become upset or discouraged. They learn that food can make them feel better or relieve their emotional sorrows. They also learn that one way to obtain extra food is to become upset and demand it.

7. Food, especially sweets, is used to reward good behavior. It may become a symbol of parental love, satisfaction, or special accomplishment.

8. The same foods are used to pacify children when they become rambunctious or bored. For parents this can be an expedient way of getting the kids out of their hair.

9. Special outings to the zoo, the park, and the movies become occasions to overindulge in fattening treats, candies, ice cream, and hot dogs. As time goes on, the outings may not be much fun without the eating (which is probably as true for many of us adults as well).

10. Nutritious but perhaps less palatable foods are made to appear as necessary evils, while rich desserts become a cause for celebration and fanfare. The underlying message is that only the rich foods should be eaten whenever the opportunity arises.

11. The net effect of all these experiences is that young children learn to eat many of the wrong foods. They also learn to consume more than they need for normal growth and activities. In the words of one popular song, they become "Junk Food Junkies."

forcing. Any time a similar problem occurs, they will probably reach for solutions that worked before—more food! In other words, *just as parents teach children, children teach parents.*

Unfortunately, they can both learn to influence each other in ways that perpetuate eating problems. As fine as both parties' intentions may be, neither benefits in the long run. However, there is always opportunity for change.

BEING FAT IS NO FUN

Contrary to popular belief, the chubby child is not necessarily healthier nor happier than his[3] thinner pals. He is often prone to more physical ailments than other children his age, not to mention the complications of developing a surplus of fat cells. Because overweight children usually eat a lot of sugary food, they are also good candidates for tooth decay and expensive dental bills as well.

From a psychological standpoint overweight children also run risks. They are frequently taunted and teased by their friends, as former fat children probably remember. They may be the victim of damaging social pressure or the recipient of embarassing nicknames such as Chubby, Tubby, Fatty, Fatso, Blimp, and Balloon. Many children are very sensitive to these attacks, especially around puberty when they become more conscious of their appearance, expand social horizons, and start dating. Instead, overweight youngsters may feel inadequate, doubt their own worth, become shy and isolate themselves from others. Ironically they may even turn to more eating for solace and comfort, especially if they have learned to use food this way in the past. One problem then compounds the others. Obviously, all of them are compelling reasons for change.

For reasons of both physical and psychological health, early recognition and treatment of overweight children are ex-

---

While we acknowledge that childhood obesity is obviously not a problem restricted to boys, to avoid repetitive and sometimes disruptive use of "he or she," we are confining ourselves to the use of the masculine pronoun.

tremely important as probably the best way to *prevent* obesity from becoming a life-long condition.

LOOKING AHEAD

What can you do as a parent to avoid the consequences of persistent overeating in your child? Like obesity in adults, childhood obesity is a complex problem that takes time and effort to treat. But effective treatment usually begins at home. What *you* do can make a difference for your youngster.

The plan for the chapter is as follows: First, we discuss the technique of pinpointing eating problems in young children, which will help you discover exactly what they are! Generally, we focus on youngsters twelve and under, a period when parental influence and many of the adverse effects of being overweight are greatest. Then some recommendations for changing your child's habits are given. At the end of the chapter we talk briefly about another childhood eating problem—one that doesn't involve overeating but rather finicky eating.

PINPOINTING EATING PROBLEMS IN YOUR CHILD

DOES YOUR CHILD HAVE A WEIGHT PROBLEM?

Some parents have overweight children but don't realize the problem exists. Others choose to do nothing about it because they feel their child is merely going through a "fat" stage which he will eventually outgrow. Thus they adopt a *laissez faire* attitude. They hope time will take care of it, and occasionally their hopes are realized. Some children elect to go on diets themselves, or they may lose weight as a result of normal growth and development. However, *in most cases* weight loss never occurs. Instead, the child continues to learn and use the same kind of habits that you yourself have been trying to change.

If you're wondering whether your child is overweight, there are two steps you can take right now. One of the easiest is to use an eye ball test—simply take a close look at your youngster. Does he have a double chin, a bulging waistline, lots of fatty tissue around the upper arms, thighs, and buttocks? If so, the child is probably overweight for his size and age.

Another step to take, especially if the first one increased your suspicion, is to arrange for an appointment with your family doctor or pediatrician. During this visit your child should undergo a thorough physical examination, because hidden physical problems can lead to weight gain and therefore need to be treated. For example, there's a slight chance that childhood obesity may be related to glandular problems such as hypothyroidism or to juvenile diabetes. A few children have what is called Prader-Willi syndrome, a rare illness characterized by an insatiable appetite and a craving for huge quantities of food. This illness is often associated with mental retardation and is believed to be caused by a neurological disturbance. In all such cases medical treatment is needed.

Despite these possibilities, *very few* obese children are overweight because of physical factors. The cause in most cases has to do with poor eating and activity habits. Too often parents and children have used physical problems as an excuse for being fat. While it is true that physical difficulties occur, they are usually the *result* or the effect of being overweight, not the cause. Nevertheless, you must know about the *possible* existence of both physical causes and complications of childhood obesity. Only in this way can the most effective treatment be provided.

Another reason for consulting your physician is to obtain professional information about the normal weight range for children of different sizes and age, as well as about proper nutrition for your child. Unlike adults, children's weight and eating habits may undergo sudden change as they grow and develop physically. Knowing what is a healthy weight can clear up parental misconceptions and unrealistic expectations; it may also reduce worry when there is no cause for alarm.

LOOK BEFORE YOU LEAP: PINPOINTING PROBLEMS

As in adult life, correcting the imbalance between overeating and underexercise is the target. If your doctor tells you your child is overweight but otherwise in good health, one of the first things you should do is take a close look at your child's eating and activity patterns. You must pinpoint what your child is doing or not doing. Perhaps the easiest way to bring the problem into focus is to use an eating diary; but instead of observing your own behavior, observe those of your child. (An eating record is provided in Appendix A; you might also want to review Chapter 3 on how the record is to be used.) Usually there are plenty of occasions for home observation—at mealtime, before and after school, in the early evening, and on the weekends.

Some children gain weight because of frequent snacking between meals on cookies, candy, ice cream, and other sweets. Unless you observe your child, you will not know whether this holds true for him as well. For other children, being overweight may be due to eating second and third helpings at the main meals. There are also studies showing that overweight children are less active than their thinner pals, but this characteristic may not be true in each and every case.

The point is this: Before children can change their habits, they must know exactly what they are. Using an eating record for a week or so is one way to gain some insight. In Table 13–2 we've listed common eating habit problems you might look for.

TABLE 13–2

Common Eating Habit Problems in Children

1. Frequent between-meal snacking, especially on rich and sugary foods.
2. "Wolfing down" meals without pausing between bites or servings.
3. Asking for second helpings and receiving them.
4. Eating in front of the TV set, in the bedroom, or in places other than the family dining area.
5. Using excessive amounts of such food garnishes as butter, margarine, mayonnaise, sour cream, and rich salad dressings.
6. Feeling compelled to clean the plate at mealtime.
7. Eating a disproportionate amount of high-calorie foods (including bread, french fries, and desserts), relative to low-calorie but more nutritious foods.
8. Eating out of boredom or when angry and upset.
9. Before bedtime snacking.
10. Not knowing about foods that make up a balanced diet, nor how to discriminate between wholesome and "fat" foods.

Once you begin to observe your child's habits more closely, he may ask what you're up to. After all, children are quick to notice any change in parent behavior. While you might be able to conduct home observations of your child without being overly conspicuous (for example, by taking "mental notes" and entering them in a diary later on), trying to be unobtrusive does not always work out as planned. The question then arises, what should you do if your child asks: "Are you spying on me?" . . . "Why are you watching me?"

One approach is to ignore these questions hoping that his inquisitiveness will wane. This method may work in the short run but in the long run it antagonizes your child and prevents *mutual* cooperation needed later on. For this reason, an honest approach is probably the best one to take. Let your child know from the beginning that you're concerned about his eating habits because you want him to develop good ones—just as you want this for yourself and other members of the family. After this, ask him if he wants to learn more about his own habits and share in the use of the diary as well. Sometimes children's resistance stems not from being observed, but rather from clumsy attempts at secrecy, nagging that accompanies observations, or guilt-producing attitudes that children are unable to help themselves ("We *have* to do this because of you and your lousy eating habits"). From the time you begin home observations until a program for change is underway, working toward mutual cooperation and goal-setting with your child is an objective to keep uppermost in your mind.

IDENTIFYING REALISTIC ALTERNATIVE BEHAVIORS

Pinpointing bad eating habits is one thing. Identifying and strengthening alternative behaviors is another. Just as you want to teach your child what *not* to do, you must help him see *what to do instead.* Thus, if Greg was not munching on sweets in front of the TV set each afternoon, what else could he do? Have you offered any suggestions? What would you like to see him doing instead? Have you sat down and discussed this with him? Similarly, if Mary plays active games with her friends only rarely, how much and how often would you like to see her doing this? The task of *realistic* goal-setting in breaking old habits is as important for children as it was for you.

Table 13-3 should be completed *after* you have gathered at least a week's information (that's 7 days in a row) by means of an "eating record." In the table you should begin developing a list of specific behaviors that you would like to change in your child. For each one you put down, specify an acceptable and realistic substitute. In some cases your goal may not be to eliminate an activity entirely. For example, to insist that your child "never" again watch TV, refrain from snacking altogether, or totally avoid sweets is hardly fair. Under these circumstances your task is to reduce the frequency of these behaviors while still encouraging appropriate alternatives. A few examples are provided in the table to get you started.

TABLE 13–3

Eating Problems and Alternatives for My Child

Problem	Alternative or Goal
Examples:	
1. Snacks between meals at least 6 times a day.	1. Reduce by 50%; limit snacks to 1 after school.
2. Eats too many sweets. Prefers foods with lots of sugar and carbohydrates.	2. Encourage eating more nutritious and less caloric sweets such as fresh fruit, vegetables, and sugarless gum.
3. Watches T.V. almost continuously from 4:00 p.m. until bedtime.	3. Reduce T.V. viewing time by 25%. Increase exercise such as taking walks, bicycle riding, and doing chores in exchange for a weekly allowance.
4. Rarely plays active sports.	4. Encourage participation in swimming, softball, and bowling on family outings. Obtain membership for my son in the local "Y," Scouts, or a community recreation program.

TABLE 13–3 *(cont.)*

Problem	Alternative or Goal
1.	1.
2.	2.
3.	3.
4.	4.
5.	5.
6.	6.
7.	7.
8.	8.
9.	9.
10.	10.

WAYS TO COLLECT BASELINE INFORMATION

After pinpointing problem behaviors, you should try to gain an even more accurate picture of how often they occur. The method for homing in on problems is similar to using an eating record except that you will want to narrow your focus to the behaviors listed in Table 3-3. This information, which is preliminary in the sense that it should be collected *before* a program of change begins, is called a *baseline.* Its purpose is to give you a starting point against which later observations can be compared. As you see, the method is essentially *self-correcting.* As long as behavior changes in the desired directions, relative to a baseline level, you know that you're doing a good job. If desired changes do not occur—that is, if the old habits continue to occur at the same rate—then clearly your approach needs to be reevaluated.

Gather baseline information for one week to ten days to get a representative picture of your child's current patterns of behavior. At first, select only one of the activities you've specified in Table 13-3 and take a baseline only on that behavior. Later you can broaden your scope to achieve additional goals and objectives. For now, there is no hurry. Starting small and setting limited goals that you can build on one step at a time make it easier for you to develop new skills and for your child to learn new habits as well.

Although there are many ways to collect baseline information, two of the most common and simple methods are: (1) to observe how often the behavior happens (the *frequency*), or (2) to measure how long the behavior lasts (the *duration*). The choice of method depends on the goals you and your child set. Before beginning a baseline, ask yourself, "Do I want a certain activity to occur more or less often, or for shorter or longer periods of time?" Your answer will help you select an appropriate recording system. For example, if your goal is to reduce the number of times your child "bugs" you for snacks before dinnertime, use a frequency tally. Count how many times the behavior happens either each day or during some period of the the day when the problem typically occurs (for example, three to six P.M.). This information can be collected by say, noting each time "bugging" behavior occurs on a small index card. Or you may stick a little piece of adhesive tape on the refrigerator door after every "bugging" episode. Use whatever method is convenient for you.

On the other hand, duration recording is used when your goal is to increase or decrease the *amount of time* spent in certain activities, such as engaging in mild exercise, active play, swimming, walking, watching TV, or eating regular meals. Consider this problem: If you wanted to slow down your child's eating at dinnertime, are you asking a "how long" or "how often" question—respectively, duration or frequency? The answer is "how long," and you could collect the information by writing down the time at which dinner eating begins and ends. The difference, in minutes, is the *duration* of the behavior.

All you really need for either frequency or duration recording is a pencil and paper, and a timepiece if a duration measure is collected. You also need to specify a rule that tells when your observations are made each day (e.g., in the morning from seven to nine o'clock, at mealtime, all day, and so forth). Recording should always be done in the same way from one day to the next to allow for meaningful comparisons over time. To watch your child for five minutes one day and two hours the next does little good, because any difference would probably be due to variations in your observation time.

GRAPHING RESULTS

As you make baseline observations, the results of your efforts can be summarized in graphic form. A graph provides an ongoing picture of your child's behavior and allows you to see more clearly what's going on. A sample graph is shown in Figure 13-1. Different days or observation periods are indicated along the horizontal line, while the amount of behavior each day is shown along the vertical line. Daily results are plotted by a series of connected dots.

As the graph shows, Frank looked for snacks nine times on day 1, seven times on day 2, eight times on day 4, three times on day 5, nine times on day 6 and so forth. Day 3 was *not* graphed because observations could not be made that day as Frank was staying at a friend's house. (Note: "missed" observation days are shown graphically by a break in the connecting line.) You might want to complete the graph by filling in the information for days 9 and 10. Frank asked for snacks five times on day 9 and nine times on day 10. Where would you put the remaining two dots? Draw them in, along with the connecting line.

As always, don't be alarmed if changes don't occur immediately. *Just because problems are not eliminated overnight does not mean that a program is failing.* Sometimes parents become discouraged because they think their efforts are not working. If they were more sensitive to gradual changes over time, which a graph can clearly show, they might avoid giving up on a program that was, in fact, producing results in the right direction. A blank graph is provided in Figure 13-2 for your use. We recommend that you collect baseline information on at least one of your child's behaviors *before* continuing on with the next section.[4]

---

[4]Sometimes the act of observing and recording behavior is sufficient to change it. For some children (but not all), knowing that their behavior is being watched closely helps; desired changes may occur without further intervention. Don't be surprised if this happens. Of course, the behavior might move in the other direction. That is okay since sometimes things could be getting worse—before they get better.

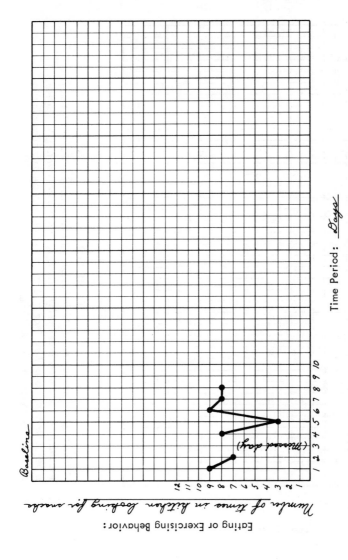

Time Period: _Days_

FIGURE 13-1

The frequency with which Frank (10 years old) is after snacks in the kitchen.

245

Eating or Exercising Behavior:

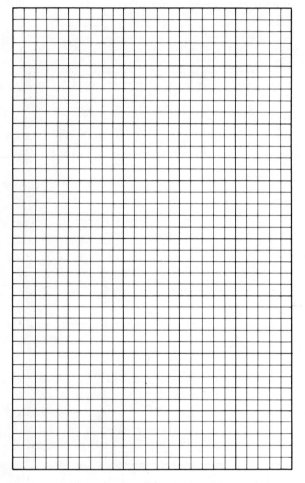

Time Period : _____

FIGURE 13-2

A blank graph. Select one of the behaviors you have listed in Table 13-3 and use this graph to collect baseline information. You will be counting how often a behavior happens or how long it lasts. Fill in the vertical axis according to the type of observation you will be using.

A POSITIVE APPROACH TO CHANGE

Once you have pinpointed problem behaviors and obtained a week or more of baseline information, you are ready to begin a program for change. As standard practice you should always inform your child of expected behaviors and enlist his cooperation in bringing them about. Too often parents fail to make their wishes and concerns known in advance. Without this information, children must rely on guesswork to meet the standards their parents set.

Your expectations should be communicated in a friendly, nonthreatening way, at a time when you have your child's undivided attention. Please, *don't demand* sweeping or unrealistic changes overnight; you'll likely only be setting up yourself and your child for disappointment later on. Avoid vague or alarmist talk in expressing your concerns. Phrases like "Why are you always so hungry . . . Your overeating has us worried to death . . . Can't you go out and play like other kids . . . You're too fat and have to stop eating so much" don't convey much useful information and only set the stage for defensiveness and resentment.

For the same reasons, nagging your child to do one thing and not another isn't very helpful either. *The atmosphere to create is one of mutual goal-setting and the cooperative pursuit of these goals.* For children (as well as for adults), habit change is easiest when it is motivated by a sense of personal commitment rather than by a fear of reprisals or persistent harassment.

Here's a dialogue between two parents and their overweight, ten-year-old son. You may get the feel for an approach.

> *Mother to her son:* Johnny, your dad and I would like to talk with you for a few minutes. Can you sit down and join us for awhile?
>
> *Child:* Now? Okay, what did you want to talk about?

Mother: After your last visit to the doctor, do you remember he told you you were too heavy, that you should lose about ten pounds? It may have sounded like he was kidding at the time, but he meant what he said. He really was concerned. Dad and I also think it would be a good idea if you took some weight off. That's what we want to discuss with you.

Dad: Losing weight isn't always easy. Take it from us, we know. But your mother and I have been helping each other lose weight for some time now, and we're getting down where we want to be. It's meant changing some old eating habits and trying to exercise more, but it's paying off. We thought you might like to join us so we can all help each other out. What do you think of that idea?

Child: Oh, I don't know. The kids tease me at school about being fat and that bugs me. I don't let them know it, but it does. I really would like to get them off my back.

Dad: If you lost the ten pounds the doctor suggested, you'd probably look much better. Do you think they'd still bug you then?

Child: Well, I don't know. I guess not. But how can I do that?

Mother: What if you were to cut out some of the in-between meal cookies and snacks. We could keep a lot of the junk foods out of the house. That might help too. We could also get out the bicycles more often and start riding again. Getting more exercise really helps. How does that sound for starters?

Child: Ah—gee. I like cookies. I don't know. I really get hungry and uh, I really like to eat something. Maybe I could stop eating those potato chips and ice cream bars at school. I know they're not very good for me.

Dad: Good idea. There are other things that are better to eat when you're trying to lose weight.

Child: Yeh, I know. Like an apple instead of the sweets.

> *Mother:* When would you like to start losing weight?
>
> *Child:* Right now.
>
> *Mother:* Good. This evening dad and I will fill you in on exactly what we've been doing. Then we can all work together.
>
> *Dad:* We're glad you want to join us, son.

As you can see, building a sense of commitment with your child, if this is at all possible, is a good way to start. On the other hand, if he is unwilling to commit himself, or if he expresses resentment or hurt at the thought of losing weight, *listen* to his reaction and try to work out a compromise plan. By all means, avoid emotional blow-ups and threats of terrible punishment for non-compliance. These reactions never help to solve problems; they can only make them worse. You should know well enough that overeating is often used to deal with the upset feelings of arguments and blow-ups.

Now that you have a general feeling for the positive atmosphere children need, you need more specific suggestions on bringing change about. Our suggested methods involve:

1. using positive consequences,
2. demonstrating how to do something (parent modeling),
3. self-observing,
4. learning to manage food better.

Each of the methods may be used alone or in combination with the others.

1. EFFECTIVE USE OF POSITIVE REINFORCEMENT

Simply stated, when your child shows the *slightest improvement,* praise him and let him know you like it. However, as was discussed in Chapter 2, some additional words of advice are needed concerning the proper use of reinforcement techniques. Following are several important considerations:

Reinforce Immediately. Practice reinforcing the desired behavior *immediately after* it occurs or at least at the time you first notice it. To give reinforcement in advance (for example, "Okay, we'll go to the show today, but next week you'll really have to cut down on your snacking."), or to wait a day or week after desired changes take place, reduces the strengthening effect of reinforcing consequences. By way of analogy, imagine you went out of your way to look radiantly beautiful for your husband—then he waited until next week to tell you he noticed. A delay in reinforcement is not only frustrating, it also makes learning a more difficult task.

Learning by Small, Gradual Steps. To expect dramatic changes in your child's behavior overnight is often unrealistic. More often these changes come about gradually and irregularly by small steps or successive approximations. For this reason, set your standards for reinforcement *low* at first, at a level that can be easily reached. We stress this because many parents have excessively high standards when it comes to their children. They expect the "best." While to expect good things is worthwhile, such views often get mixed up with how to help the child change. Help your child succeed by taking one step at a time. Obviously, reinforcing consequences can't work unless they're experienced, and they won't be experienced if the standards or expectations you set are too high. With time and patience, standards can be *increased gradually* until you have reached your final goal.

For example, if you want to help your child slow down his eating or strengthen his preference for less fattening foods, you should start by reinforcing the *slightest* change toward these goals. In some cases a few seconds difference or even a small bite of nonpreferred but nutritious food should be acknowledged with pleasant attention. The same holds true for changing exercise habits or reducing between meal snacks. *Any improvement* is at least a step in the right direction, and it makes the next step easier.

Both gradual learning and effective encouragement of behavior rely heavily on accurate baseline information, for improvement is gauged against this standard.

How Often Should You Reinforce?: Schedules. Scheduling refers to how often reinforcers are given: you can reinforce each time a behavior occurs, once at some time of the day, and after certain number of occurrences; and so on. Reinforcing consequences can be given according to many different schedules. But since different schedules influence behavior in different ways, deciding on a schedule requires some thinking on your part. The decision should not be left to guesswork or intuition alone.

Beginning a program, give reinforcers frequently and continuously—in other words, as often as you can. Frequent reinforcement helps to motivate your child quickly and strengthen his commitment; it also builds behavior when you are moving from one approximation to the next. After the program is well under way and desired changes are occurring consistently, you can gradually reduce the amount of reinforcement; that is, you can move from continuous reinforcement (each time or nearly every time the behavior happens) to reinforcement on a more *intermittent* basis (every so often). One of the nice things about intermittent reinforcement is that it helps to keep behavior going and makes it more resistant to change. Occasional rewards have the effect of maintaining behavior for a long time.

Set the rate of movement from continuous to intermittent reinforcement according to the information you're collecting. If progress slows or your child's behavior reverts to baseline level—graphing your results regularly will show you either—you may be "thinning" your schedule of reinforcement too fast. If so, slow down and be more patient. Providing liberal doses of good things is more important than jeopardizing the progress you and your child have made.

What Are Some Reinforcers to Use?: Choice. Many different types of reinforcing consequence are available to you. Probably the best is *praise,* or expressions of positive attention and approval. For most parents praise is fairly easy to give, and it's a natural part of parent-child relations as well. However, be selective in what you praise, making sure that it's consistent with your goals. Rewarding your child for leaving food on his plate at home, while praising him for eating two helpings when you visit the in-laws, does little good.

One way to remind yourself to praise progress frequently and correctly is to display your graph in a conspicuous place for you as well as for your youngster. Allowing your child to decorate or design his graph and to carry out his own charting can also be a helpful approach. Seeing positive results is not only highly rewarding in its own right, but it also helps to build a sense of self-mastery and better self-esteem.

Finally praise and social approval must be expressed in a *sincere* way. Both can backfire if done so mechanically ("That's a good boy. Very good, very good . . ."), so matter-of-factly, or so effusively that it comes across as phony. Praise is not meant to be used, as a "sugar coated pill," to entice behavior you know will be unpleasant. Instead, it should be offered in a genuine way and accompanied by the appropriate tone of voice, facial expression, eye contact, and physical contact. You may understandably feel a little awkward and self-conscious about praising your child if you have not been doing it very often. The point is that you must mean it and be sincere in offering the praise.

In addition to praise, another type of reinforcer includes access to certain events and activities. For example, bike rides, games, watching TV, story telling, allowances, or special outings are all naturally occurring reinforcers that can be made available *after* some desired behavior change or weight loss occurs. Some people have referred to this principle as "Grandma's Law," meaning that preferred activities occur only *after* less preferred ones take place: for example, "Straighten your room up and then you may go out and play . . . Lose two pounds this week and then we will add an extra fifty cents to your weekly allowance." This approach not only motivates behavior, but it also teaches the child to delay his gratification for pleasurable events.

Some parents prefer to use points, stars, or other *tokens* as rewarding consequences.[5] These can be given immediately after desired activities occur—a distinct advantage in many cases— then exchanged later for other rewards in the same way that we exchange money for various commodities.

If you elect to use a point or token system, it's important to explain to your child *in advance:* (1) exactly how he can earn tokens, (2) what he can exchange them for, (3) how many tokens he needs to complete the exchange, and (4) when the exchange takes place. For example, in Figure 13–1 the problem of asking for too many between-meal snacks could have been approached indirectly by reinforcing other alternative behaviors, such as completing household chores, with points. As long as the alternative behaviors produce nice consequences, they will occur, and the motivation to hang around the kitchen will be correspondingly reduced. After all, hunting for snacks and doing chores in other parts of the house can't very well occur at the same time. Remember, though, that points themselves have no intrinsic value; they are only symbols of progress toward some other "back-up" reinforcer. After a certain number of points are accumulated (not too many—remember the step-by-step principle), they can be exchanged for a toy airplane, a trip to the movies, or something else the child desires.

To see how the results of a "point program" look in graphic form, refer to Figure 13–3. Would you say the program is working? The rather sudden and consistent reduction in asking for snacks, after the points were made available for other activities, suggests that it is.

[5]For additional information on token reinforcement systems you might want to consult W. Becker's book, *Parents are Teachers,* or G. Patterson's book, *Families.*

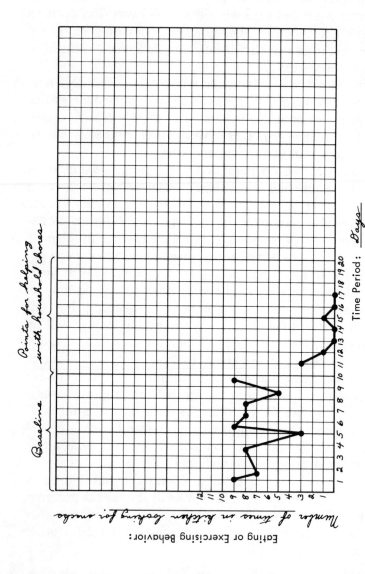

FIGURE 13-3

The frequency with which Frank (10 years old) is after snacks in the kitchen before and after points were given for helping with household chores.

Identifying effective reinforcers and using them systematically to gradually build and maintain desired behavior is the essence of positive reinforcement. In Table 13–4 list as many reinforcing events and activities for your child as you can. Although expressions of praise, encouragement, and affection are almost always appropriate, what other things might increase your child's motivation? If you think for a while, you'll probably come up with quite a few. *Why not ask your youngster for suggestions?* After all, he probably knows best what he likes and dislikes.

TABLE 13–4
Possible Reinforcers for My Child

Examples:

1. Weekly allowance
2. Going to bed a half hour later in the evening.
3. A trip to the movies, the park, the zoo, etc.
4. Storytelling
5. Barbie doll clothes.

1.

2.

3.

4.

5.

6.

7.

8.

9.

10.

2. POSITIVE PARENT MODELING

At one time or another all of us learn by observing others and then trying out what we've observed. For children this process is especially applicable: They are inclined to adopt many of the behaviors they see their parents doing. For this reason you should model behaviors that you want to strengthen in your child; then reinforce them when they occur.

For example, if you want to encourage your child to exercise more, you might begin a series of daily calisthenics or participate in some family sports such as the ones described in Chapter 6. As you model the behavior, your child might elect to join in spontaneously or you could ask if he'd like to accompany you. Of if you want to see your child snacking less, eating slower, eating more nutritious and less caloric foods, ask yourself if you're modeling good behaviors for him. If not, become a positive model instead. Again the saying "Do as I say, not as I do" is relevant. Parents often do not realize that their actions can easily override the impact of their words, because children are such excellent observers! Saying *and* doing what you say is a powerful combination.

3. SELF-OBSERVING

Earlier *your* keeping an eating diary for your child was pointed out to be a good way to learn where problems exist and what changes need to be made. Children at the grade school level and above, however, should be able to observe their own behavior in much the same way. You might encourage your child to keep an eating or activity diary himself and in the process he may become more aware of his own behavior. Instruction on how to self-observe can be given in a friendly, helping way that need not imply parental displeasure or alarm.

As you know, the technique itself is fairly straightforward and requires only that you spell out which behaviors need to be recorded. Your child might keep either a comprehensive eating record (such as the one described in Chapter 3) or keep a record of events such as the type and number of between-meal snacks, foods eaten at school, or exercise engaged in each day. In either case, if you ask your child to collect this information, remember to reinforce him when he does. As always, start out slowly and don't ask him to observe too much.

Self-observing is a useful way to help children acquire better *self-control*. Studies have shown that asking children to jot down what they do enables them to study better in the classroom, to reduce disruptions such as talking out or roaming around without the teacher's permission, even to brush their teeth more regularly. In the same way it can help your child correct bad eating habits that may affect his health and weight.

However, there are other benefits of self-observing. For one, you can use the information your child provides to gauge his progress away from home and to gradually build improvements as they occur. The same information can also be used to teach your child facts about proper nutrition. For example, once you have a better idea of what your child is eating, you can teach him how to distinguish high- from low-calorie foods, or nutritiously valuable foods from those that are mainly sugar and carbohydrate. Knowing which foods make up a well- balanced diet is important if children are to learn to make proper choices regarding food. Finally, the act of self-observing can serve as a constant reminder for children to engage in appropriate behaviors even when parents or other authority figures are not around. To the extent that these behaviors happen, your child will be learning a valuable lesson in self-control. In the long run, that is the objective you want to achieve.

4. HELPING YOUR CHILD MANAGE FOOD BETTER

As you learned earlier, much of our eating behavior is influenced by what happens around us, by environmental cues. One way to facilitate weight loss is to rearrange your home (including social) surroundings so the temptation to overeat is reduced. The same principles hold true for children's weight problems, and a review of them should suffice.

Too Many Fattening Foods.   Curbing your child's consumption of fattening foods can be accomplished by not purchasing them, or at least by not leaving them conspicuously placed around the house. In place of high-caloric snacks, keep a rich supply of carrot sticks, celery, or fresh fruit in places where they are readily accessible.

Overeating at Mealtime.   Overeating at mealtime can also be reduced by preparing and serving smaller portions of food, keeping extra food in the kitchen instead of on the table, avoiding problem foods during regular meals, and experimenting with tasty alternatives to rich desserts. Such alternatives may be jello, fresh fruit, dietetic puddings and cola, dried fruit, popsicles made from fruit juice. In the process of eating, you can model eating slowly, pausing between bites, putting your utensils down when eating, and chewing your food thoroughly. Showing your child better ways to eat food helps to get new habits started. By praising him for specific actions (such as eating more slowly) you can keep him trying to improve.

Breaking Up Associations Between Eating and Other Activities.   To break up old associations between eating and such activities as TV viewing, bedtime, sitting in the playroom, the number of eating situations can be narrowed. For example, eating can be limited to the dining area only. In place of eating you might also encourage a gradual exercise program, such as the one you may have started. Why not ask your child to join in? Better yet, walks, bike expeditions, trips to the swimming pool, and other enjoyable forms of physical exercise can become family affairs planned to occur on a more regular basis than they have been in the past.

What Does Your Child Know About Food? An important step toward better food management is nutritional counseling. Just as you have probably helped your child learn to count, spell, read, or tell time, you can also help him learn the nutritional value of various foods and the type of food groups that make up a balanced diet. (Refer to Chapter 5 for a discussion of proper nutrition and food exchange diets.) Having your child help you prepare the shopping list is not out of the question either, so request his assistance in preparing the family meals. By so doing, you give your youngster a chance to put his knowledge to use and the occasion to determine what he eats; you can also check on the adequacy of his suggestions and provide corrective feedback if necessary. However, before corrective feedback can be given, make sure your knowledge is in fact *correct*. In many cases parents themselves need to be better informed about basic food groups, calories, proteins, minerals, and vitamins. Otherwise only misinformation is communicated.

WHAT TO DO ABOUT FINICKY EATING

A discussion of children's eating problems would be incomplete without some mention of finicky eating. Virtually all parents have heard their child say at one time or another, ''Not that again. I don't want any.'' The infamous battle cry of children—''Yuk''—has a way of discrediting the attraction of many foods and of signaling a hasty retreat from the table with a staunch refusal to eat. The problem here is certainly not to cut back overeating so much as to encourage eating certain foods, especially those that are nonpreferred but nutritiously valuable. Incidentally, though not an unusual or serious problem if it occurs only on rare occasions, finicky eating can become a significant problem when it becomes a nightly occurrence and serves as a source of continuous friction between parent and child.

Parents frequently coax, threaten, nag, or otherwise pressure their child to eat. While these methods sometimes produce a momentary victory, the fact that finicky eating returns during subsequent meals underscores its long-run ineffectiveness. Parental attempts to force eating may have the effect of reinforcing just the opposite behavior. Under these conditions exploring alternative approaches is imperative. Here are a few, many of which are based on principles you've already discovered.

Prepare Interesting Dishes.   Experiment with novel ways of serving and preparing meals to increase the attractiveness of food for your child. Instead of serving large portions of preferred foods only, while avoiding nonpreferred foods altogether, try serving mini portions of a nutritionally balanced meal. As your child samples new foods, praise him for doing so. Later on you can gradually increase the size of his serving. Certain difficult foods, such as salads or vegetables, can sometimes be made more palatable by preparing them to resemble a clown's face, a bunny rabbit, or some other interesting object.

By the way, don't be alarmed if your child doesn't eat all his meat and vegetables or fails to drink three glasses of milk each day. If he eats a range of foods, he's not going to suffer from malnutrition or experience a vitamin deficiency by occasional finicky behavior.

Use Natural Reinforcers To Encourage Better Eating. Natural reinforcers, such as dessert or other preferred foods,

can be offered *after* your child has tried a little of a new food—
another example of "Grandma's Law." On the other hand, because refraining from argumentative power struggles with your
child over what and how much he *must* eat is best, try ignoring
your child's complaints rather than hooking in.

Positive Modeling. Be a positive model for your child and eat
a variety of foods, but don't insist that he eat every food, after
all, you don't like everything either. Also avoid threatening
your child or justifying his finickiness. Phrases such as,
"Won't you eat a little more for your mother? . . . You won't
grow big and strong if you don't eat . . . I know you won't like
this but eat it anyway . . . Daddy didn't like it when he was little either" usually aren't very helpful. They may elicit a little
guilt or bring about begrudging compliance, but in the long run
they don't produce lasting behavior change.

GETTING IT ALL TOGETHER.[6]

Hopefully this chapter has provided you with useful information on how to change your child's eating and exercise
habits. To assess your progress, check the list below. Answer
each question quickly and honestly.

1. Have you carefully read the section on "Facts About
   Childhood Obesity," including Table 13-1, "How
   Children Learn to Overeat"? Yes_____ No_____

[6]*A cautionary note:* Sometimes a chronic refusal to eat is a sign of
serious psychological disturbance. For example, there is an illness called
anorexia nervosa that is characterized by a generalized aversion to food and
severe weight loss (as high as forty percent of normal body weight). This condition is usually found in females during adolescence or young adulthood and
sometimes follows a starvation or crash diet which simply doesn't stop. If you
suspect this problem in your family, contact your doctor at once.

2. Have you talked with your pediatrician or physician to determine if your child is overweight for his size and age, and whether this might be due to physical causes? Yes_____ No_____

3. Have you observed your child carefully (by means of an eating record) to pinpoint potential eating habit problems and to discover more acceptable alternative behaviors? Yes_____ No_____

4. Have you come up with an appropriate measurement system by which habit change can be assessed? Yes_____ No_____

5. Have you taken a week or more of baseline information on each of the problems you've listed? Yes_____ No_____

6. Have you been graphing the results of your efforts? Yes_____ No_____

7. Have you discussed problem areas with your child to identify mutually agreed-upon goals and to obtain his cooperation in bringing them about? Yes_____ No_____

8. Have you identified appropriate rewards you can use to motivate your child? Yes _____ No_____

9. Are you remembering to watch your child when he's good and to praise him for improvement? Yes_____ No_____

10. Have you broken down your goals into a series of small gradual steps to help your child succeed? Yes_____ No_____

11. Have you continued to monitor progress *after* a program for change was instituted? Yes_____ No_____

12. Have you asked your child to begin observing his own eating and exercise habits, then praising him when he does? Yes_____ No_____

13. Are you helping your child manage food better by keeping "junk" foods out of the house, serving smaller portions of food, and narrowing the conditions under which eating occurs? Yes_____ No_____

14. Have you talked with your child about proper nutrition, and did he understand what you said? Yes_____ No_____

15. Are you remembering to be patient with your child? As we've emphasized repeatedly, improvement will come but it takes time. Yes_____ No_____

If your were able to answer "yes" to most of these questions, congratulate yourself and your child. Keep up the good work and your child will be on the road to keeping off those extra pounds permanently. If you answered "no" to a number of questions, go back to those questions and figure out what the problem might be. Re-read the relevant section in Chapter 13, even re-read appropriate chapters in the book, as these can help you implement a better weight loss program with your child. Experiment and keep trying until you find things that work for your child.

There are no easy ways to reduce or to maintain your ideal weight. Managing your weight is a lifelong process. By consistently using the principles in this book, they will become part of your life, and you and your child will take off and keep off those excess pounds.

Appendix **A**

Eating Record

Day _____
Date _____

Time:	Food			Place: Home, Work, Restaurant	People: Alone, Family Friends	Hunger and Feelings
Start/Stop	Quantity	Type	Calories			

Eating Record

Day ————
Date ————

Time:	Food			Place: Home, Work, Restaurant	People: Alone, Family Friends	Hunger and Feelings
Start/Stop	Quantity	Type	Calories			

Eating Record

Time:	Food			Place: Home, Work, Restaurant	People: Alone, Family Friends	Hunger and Feelings
Start/Stop	Quantity	Type	Calories			

Eating Record

Day _____

Date _____

Time:	Food			Place: Home, Work, Restaurant	People: Alone, Family Friends	Hunger and Feelings
Start/Stop	Quantity	Type	Calories			

Day _____
Date _____

Time		Food			Place Home, Work, Restaurant	Persons Alone, Family, Friends	Hunger None, Feelings	Change
Start	Finish	Quantity	Type	Calories				

Eating Record

Day _____
Date _____

Time:	Food			Place: Home, Work, Restaurant	People: Alone, Family Friends	Hunger and Feelings
Start/Stop	Quantity	Type	Calories			

Food Measurements

Weight		*Metric System*
16 ounces (oz.)	1 ounce = 1 pound (lb.)	=28.35 grams (gm.) =0.45 kilograms
Volume		
3 teaspoons (tsp.) 2 tablespoons (tbs.) 1 cup 1 quart (qt.)	1 teaspoon = 1 tablespoon = 1 fluid ounce (fl. oz.) = 1/2 pint (pt.) = 16 tablespoons = 2 pints (pt.) = 4 cups = 8 fluid ounces	= 5 milliliters (ml.) = 15 milliliters = 30 milliliters = .24 liters (l.) = .96 liters
Length		
	1 inch (in.)	= 2.5 centimeters (cm.)

Appendix

Food Measurements

Appendix C

Seven Day Menu Plan*

Day 1

Breakfast	Calories	Total Calories
Orange—1-2½ " sliced	65	
Poached egg—1 large	80	
Whole wheat toast—1 slice	60	
Butter—1/3 tbs.	35	
Coffee or tea	—	
		240

Lunch		
Tomato juice—½ cup	25	
Toasted cheese sandwich		
Whole wheat bread—1 slice	60	
Cheddar cheese—2 oz.	230	
Applesauce unsweetened—½ cup	50	
Coffee or tea	—	
		365

Day 1 (*cont.*)

Dinner	Calories	Total Calories
Rice (instant cooked)—½ cup	105	
*Steak terriaki	268	
Chinese pods & mushrooms (boiled)		
4 oz. serving	70	
Canned dietetic fruit cocktail		
4 oz. serving-water packed	42	
Coffee or tea	—	
		485
Total Calories for Day		1,090

Steak Terriaki
  3/4 lbs. flank steak (thin slices)
  Onion—1/3 medium chopped
  Ginger—1½ tsp. powdered
  Sherry—½ cup
  Soy Sauce—1 cup
  1/3 tbs. sugar
  1 large clove garlic chopped

Combine all ingredients except steak and mix
well. Add steak slices and marinate for two
hours or more in refrigerator. Cook quickly
on both sides in broiler or over charcoal. Serves
two.

*These menus range from 1,000 to 1,200 calories per day. If your meal plan calls for
more than 1,200 calories per day, you may add a little food to these menus. We thank
Rashel Jeffrey for writing and testing these menus.

Day 2

Breakfast	Calories	Total Calories
Orange juice—4 oz.	60	
Oatmeal—3/4 cup	130	
Skim milk—1/2 cup	45	
Coffee	—	

Day 2 (*cont.*)

Breakfast	*Calories*	*Total Calories*
Lunch		

Cottage cheese w/vegetables		
Cottage cheese (uncreamed) ½ cup	85	
Tomato—1-2½ ″ in diameter, sliced	25	
Scallion—1 chopped	3	
Cucumber—½ pared, diced	10	
Radishes—2 medium	2	
Salt & pepper	—	
Roll—½ hard	78	
Butter—½ teaspoon or 1/3 ″ thick pat	18	
Skim milk—1 cup	90	
		311

Dinner		
*Broiled halibut steak brushed with ½ pat butter (margarine) and lemon slice—4 oz.	214	
Small baked potato with 1 pat butter (margarine)	125	
Green beans—½ cup	17	
Strawberries . ½ cup	30	
Half & half cream—¼ cup	82	
Coffee or tea	—	
Artificial sweetener	—	
		468
Total Calories for Day		1,014

*Brush Halibut steak with butter on both sides and season with salt and pepper. broil each side about six minutes or until fish flakes when pressed with a fork. Serve with a lemon slice. Serves two.

Day 3

Breakfast	*Calories*	*Total Calories*

Grapefruit juice—4 oz., canned, unsweetened	50	
Scrambled egg—1, milk and fat	110	
English muffin—½	70	
Butter—½ pat	18	

Day 3 (*cont.*)

Breakfast	Calories	Total Calories
Coffee or tea	—	
		248

Lunch		
Open-faced Sandwich		
Rye bread—1 slice	60	
Mayonnaise—1 tsp.	33	
White meat, chicken—2 oz.	120	
Swiss cheese, natural—1 ″ cube	55	
Lettuce—1 wedge, 1/6 head	10	
Fresh cherries—½ cup	41	
Skim milk—1 cup	90	
		409

Dinner		
Vegetable juice cocktail—3/4 cup	31	
*Fish with vegetables	350	
Boiled potatoes served with		
parsley and 1 pat butter	70	
Dietetic pineapple slices—½ cup	44	
Coffee or tea	—	495
Total Calories for Day		1,152

*Fish with Vegetables
1# Fresh or frozen flounder
2 tbs. butter or margarine
1 tbs. white wine
16 oz. canned tomatoes, drained—save half
   the juice
Lemon, to taste
Salt and pepper and garlic salt, to taste
3 Carrots, peeled and diced
1 Onion, peeled and sliced
1 Green pepper, sliced

Place fish in baking dish, add lemon juice, salt,
pepper and garlic salt, and vegetables. Cover
with canned tomatoes and wine. Bake covered
at 350° for forty minutes or until fish flakes
and vegetables are tender. Serves 2.

Day 4

Breakfast	Calories	Total Calories
Corn flakes—1-1/6 cup	110	
Blueberries—½ cup	45	
Skim milk—½ cup	45	
Coffee or tea	—	
		200

Lunch

	Calories	Total Calories
Beef patty—3 oz.	185	
Hamburger roll—½	60	
Cottage cheese—½ cup uncreamed	85	
Peaches dietetic—½ cup	40	
Coffee or tea	—	
		370

Dinner

	Calories	Total Calories
*Chicken cacciatore—1 serving	224	
Rice (cooked, instant)—½ cup	76	
Salad—small tossed	20	
2 leaves lettuce		
½ sliced cucumber		
½ sliced tomato		
Italian dressing (low calorie)— tbs. 10		
Melon balls—1 cup with lime juice	43	
Coffee or tea	—	
		363
Total Calories for Day		933

*Chicken cacciatore
2 Skinned chicken breasts (4 oz.)
½ Onion, chopped
2 tbs. corn oil
½ Bay leaf
¼ teaspoon garlic salt
⅛ teaspoon Oregano
4 oz. tomato juice
2 tbs. ketchup mixed with 2 tbs. water
Salt and pepper to taste

In large sauce pan saute onion in oil. Salt and pepper chicken breasts, place in pan and brown on both sides. Combine other ingredients and pour in pan. Simmer covered for one hour. Serves two.

Day 5

Breakfast	Calories	Total Calories
Grapefruit—½ cup sections	40	
Rye toast—1 slice	60	
Butter—1 sq. in. pat	35	
Hard cheese—1 cube	65	
Coffee or tea	—	
		200

Lunch		
Chef salad		
Chef salad dressing—1 tbs.	16	
Hard boiled egg—½ large	40	
Chicken-sliced thin, 1 oz.	60	
Boiled ham-sliced thin, 1 oz.	68	
American cheese—½ oz.	53	
Tomato—1-2½ " diameter	33	
Cucumber—½ pared	10	
Carrot—½ cup sliced	27	
Lettuce—2 large leaves	5	
Rye crisp crackers—4	68	
Coffee or tea	—	
		380

Dinner		
*Hot crab puffs—1 serving	142	
Stewed tomatoes—1 cup	72	
Corn on the cob with one pat		
butter or margarine—1 ear	105	
Honeydew melon with blueberries—		
1 slice 2" × 7"	45	
Coffee or tea	—	364
Total Calories for Day		944

*Hot Crab Puffs

1 English muffin, divided in half
Lemon and parsley
Combine:
One third can (3 oz.) crabmeat cleaned and
  drained
One sixth medium onion, chopped

Day 5 (*cont.*)

Breakfast	Calories	Total Calories

One eighth cup mayonnaise
One eighth cup chopped celery
Three fourth teaspoon lemon juice
One third ounce cheddar cheese shredded

Spread crab mixture on each half of English muffin. Broil for about two minutes under broiler (until cheese melts). Garnish with lemon slices and parsley. Serves two.

Day 6

Breakfast	Calories	Total Calories
Apple juice—½ cup	60	
Raisin Bran cereal—3/5 cup	100	
Skim milk—½ cup	45	
Cantaloupe—one fourth medium	30	
Coffee or tea	—	
		235

Lunch	Calories	Total Calories
Shrimp salad		
Small can shrimp—3 oz.	100	
Lettuce wedge—1/6 head	10	
Hard boiled egg—1 large	80	
Celery—3" to 5" stalks	10	
Lemon juice—1 tbs.	4	
Grapes—small bunch	55	
Italian bread—1 slice, .8 oz.	65	
Coffee or tea	—	
		324

Dinner	Calories	Total Calories
Tomato juice—½ cup	25	
*Veal with herbs—1 chop approx.	380	
Noodles—½ cup	100	
*Glazed carrots	40	

Day 6 (*cont.*)

Breakfast	Calories	Total Calories
*Baked pear	35	
Coffee or tea	—	
		580
Total Calories for Day		1,139

*Veal with Herbs
2 Veal chops—1″ thick, trimmed
1/6 cup corn oil
Salt and pepper
1/3 clove garlic
1/3 small onion, sliced
1/3 cup dry white wine
1/6 tsp. parsley, tarragon, thyme (combined)
1/3 beef bullion
1/6 cup water

Saute onion and garlic in oil. Add veal and
quickly brown on both sides. Add remaining
ingredients. Cover, simmer slowly for twenty
mins. Serves two.

*Glazed Carrots
3/4 cups sliced carrots, simmered in just
enough water to cover, till tender. Add 1
tablespoon honey. Simmer until the liquid
evaporates. Serves two.

*Baked Pears
Warm 1/3 can of pears with 1/8 teaspoon
ginger and slice of lemon.

Day 7

Breakfast	Calories	Total Calories
Apricot juice—4 oz.	60	
*Scrambled egg—1 large	100	
White bread—1 thin slice	55	
Coffee or tea	—	

*Add herbs—½ tsp. parsley, chives, tarragon,
  combined. Add milk.   215

Day 7 *(cont.)*

Breakfast	*Calories*	*Total Calories*

Lunch

Salmon salad		
Canned salmon—3 oz.	189	
Lemon Juice—1 tsp.	4	
Chopped onion—1 tsp.	4	
Mayonnaise—1 tsp.	33	
Lettuce—¼ head ⁻	15	
Crackers—4 1-7/8″ saltines	50	
Cantaloupe—¼ of 5 ″	30	
Coffee or tea	—	
		325

Dinner

*Beef consomme—1 cup	50	
Roast pork-lean—4 oz.	277	
Mashed potatoes, milk added—½ cup	70	
*Lemony zucchini	84	
Lettuce—2 large leaves	5	
Baked apple with lemon juice, artificial sweetener and ginger	80	
Coffee or tea	—	
		566
Total Calories for Day		1,106

Beef Consommé (to spice up canned
consomme)
Add one bay leaf and a little sherry to a can
of beef consommé. Heat and serve. Simmer
to reduce liquid.

Lemony Zucchini
2 medium zucchini
3/8 cup water
1/4 cup chopped parsley
1/16 cup margarine
1/2 tablespoon minced onion
1/8 teaspoon fresh grated lemon peel
1 tablespoon fresh lemon juice
Combine all ingredients. Cook in covered
skillet until tender. Serves two.

Snacks

	The daily menus leave room for a few snacks, such as the following;
Fruits	Apple—80 calories
	Banana—85 calories
	Peach—30 calories
	Watermelon (wedge)—110 calories
Popcorn	1 cup, cooked with oil and salt added—41 calories
Pickles	1 dill—15 calories
Raw Vegetables	Celery
	Carrots
	Radishes
	Other raw vegetables

Appendix **D**

Summary Food Exchange Lists

SUMMARY FOOD EXCHANGE LISTS

1. Vegetable Exchanges	2. Fruit Exchanges	3. Bread Exchanges	4. Meat/Protein Exchanges
Raw, Any Amount	**40 Calories**	**70 Calories**	**75 Calories**
Celery	Apple Juice, 1/3 c.	*Breads*	Beef, 1 oz.
Chicory	Apple, 1 small	Bread, 1 slice	Lamb, 1 oz.
Chinese Cabbage	Applesauce, 1/2 c.	Bagel, small, 1/2	Pork, 1 oz.
Endive	Apricots, 2 medium	**Biscuit, 1**	Veal, 1 oz.
Escarole	Apricot Juice, 1/2 c.	Cornbread, 1 1/2 in.	Poultry, 1 oz.
Green Pepper	Banana, 1/2 small	Dressings, 1/3 c.	**Fish: Any fresh or frozen, 1 oz.**
Lettuce	Berries, 1 c.	Flour, 2 1/2 tbs.	Salmon, Tuna, Mackerel, 1/4 c.
Parsley	Cantaloupe, 1/4	Hamburger Bun, 1/2	Crab and Lobster, 1/4 c.
Radishes	Cherries, 10	Hot Dog Bun, 3/4	Clams, Oysters, Scallops,
Watercress	Cherry Juice, 1/2 c.	Muffin, small, 1/2	Shrimp, 1
	Dates, 2	Roll, 1	Sardines, 3
25 Calories, one half cup	Figs, dried, 2	Tortilla, 1	
Asparagus	Fruit Cocktail, 1/2 c.		Protein Substitutes
Bean Sprouts	Grapefruit, 1/2 small	*Cereals*	Cheese, 1 oz.
Beets	Grapefruit Juice, 1/2 c.	Cereal, cooked, 1/2 c.	Cottage Cheese, 1/4 c.
Broccoli	Grapes, small, 12	Cereal, dry, 3/4 c.	Dried Beans & Peas, 1/2 c.
Brussel Sprouts	Grape Juice, 1/4 c.	Grits, 1/2 c.	Peanut Butter, 2 tbs.
Cabbage	Honeydew Melon, 1/3	Rice, 1/2 c.	
Carrots	Nectarines, 1 medium	Spaghetti, noodles, pasta,	
Cauliflower	Orange, 1	1/2 c.	
Cucumbers	Orange Juice, 1/2 c.	Wheat Germ, 1/4 c.	
Eggplant	Peach, 1 medium		
Greens	Peach Juice, 1/2 c.	*Crackers*	
Chard	Pear, 1 small	Graham, 2	
Collard	Pineapple, 1/2 c.	Matzoth, 1/2	
Dandelion	Pineapple Juice, 1/2 c.	Oyster, 20	
Kale	Plums, 2	Round, 6	
Mustard	Prunes, dried, 2	Ry Krisp, 6	
Spinach	Raisins, 2 tbs.	Saltines, 5	
Turnip	Tangerine, 1	Soda, 3	
Mushrooms	Tangerine Juice, 1/2 c.		
Okra	Watermelon, 1 small slice	*Vegetables*	
Onions		Beans, dried, 1/2 c.	
Rhubarb		Corn, 1/3 c.	
Rutabaga		Corn, popped, 1 c.	
Sauerkraut		Peas, 1/2 c.	
Stringbeans,		Potato, baked, 1	
green or yellow		Potato, mashed, 1/2 c.	
Summer Squash		Pumpkin, 3/4 *c.*	
Tomatoes		Winter Squash, 1/2 c.	
Turnips		Yam, 1/2 c.	
Vegetable Juice Cocktail			
Zucchini			

5. Milk Exchanges	6. High-Calorie Food Exchanges	
80 Calories	**45 Calories**	
Non-Fat Fortified	6A. *Fats*	
Skim Milk, 1 c.		
Canned, evaporated skim, 1/2 c.	*Polyunsaturated Fats*	*Saturated Fats*
Powered (Non-Fat Dry), 1/3 c.	Margarine, soft, tub or	Margarine, regular stick, 1 tsp.
	stick, 1 t.	
Buttermilk, skimmed, 1 c.	Avocado (4 ' in diameter), 1/8	Butter, 1 tsp.
Yogurt, Skimmed Plain, 1 c.	Oil, Corn, Cottonseed,	Bacon fat, 1 tsp.
	Safflower, Soy, Sunflower,	
	1 tsp.	Bacon, crisp, 1 strip
Low-Fat Fortified	Oil, Olive, 1 tsp.	Cream, light, 2 tbs.
2% Fat Fortified Milk, 3/4 c.	Oil, Peanut, 1 tsp.	Cream, sour, 2 tbs.
2% Yogurt, plain, 3/4 c.	Olives, 5 small	Cream, heavy, 1 tbs.
	Almonds, 10 whole	Cream Cheese, 1 tbs.
Whole Milk	Pecans, 2 large whole	French dressing, 1 tbs.
Whole Milk, 1/2 c.	Peanuts, Spanish, 20 whole	Italian dressing, 1 tbs.
Buttermilk, 1/2 c.	Peanuts, Virginia, 100 whole	Lard, 1 tsp.
Yogurt, Plain, 1/2 c.	Walnuts, 6 small	Mayonnaise, 1 tsp.
	Nuts, other, 6 small	Salad dressing, mayonnaise
		type, 2 tsp.
		Salt Pork, 3/4 " cube

SUMMARY FOOD EXCHANGE LISTS (Cont.)

7. No Calorie Exchanges

	6B. *Sweets*	6C. *Beverages*
Boullion		
Clear Broth	Cake, without icing, 1"	Beer, 4 oz.
Coffee	Cake, with icing, 1/2"	Carbonated Beverage
Cranberries	Candy, 1/2 oz.	(e.g. coke), 4 oz.
Gelatin	Jam or Jelly, 1 tbs.	Liquor, 1/2 oz., 1/3 jigger
Horseradish	Pie, 1" piece of small pie	Wine, dry, 12%, 2 oz.
Lemon	Sugar or Honey, 1 tbs.	Wine, sweet, 1 oz.
Low-Calorie Soft Drinks	Syrup, 1 tbs.	
Mustard		
Pepper		
Pickle		
Rennet Tablets		
Saccharin		
Seasonings		
Spices		
Tea		
Vinegar		

Appendix **E**

Weekley Caloric Intake Diaries

1,000-Calorie Food Plan/Weekly Caloric Intake Diary

	Monday B / L / D / S	Tuesday B / L / D / S	Wednesday B / L / D / S	Thursday B / L / D / S	Friday B / L / D / S	Saturday B / L / D / S	Sunday B / L / D / S
1. Vegetable Exchanges A any amount B 25 calories	A A ○ ○	A A ○ ○	A A ○ ○	A A ○ ○	A A ○ ○	A A ○ ○	A A ○ ○
2. Fruit Exchanges 40 calories	○ ○ ○	○ ○ ○	○ ○ ○	○ ○ ○	○ ○ ○	○ ○ ○	○ ○ ○
3. Bread Exchanges 70 calories	○ ○ ○	○ ○ ○	○ ○ ○	○ ○ ○	○ ○ ○	○ ○ ○	○ ○ ○
4. Meat Exchanges 75 calories	○ ○ ○ ○	○ ○ ○ ○	○ ○ ○ ○	○ ○ ○ ○	○ ○ ○ ○	○ ○ ○ ○	○ ○ ○ ○
5. Milk Exchanges 80 calories	○ ○	○ ○	○ ○	○ ○	○ ○	○ ○	○ ○
6. Fats, Sweets and Beverages Exchanges 45 calories	○ ○ ○	○ ○ ○	○ ○ ○	○ ○ ○	○ ○ ○	○ ○ ○	○ ○ ○
7. Unlimited Exchanges 0 calories	A A	A A	A A	A A	A A	A A	A A
Food Exchange Calories							
Additional Calories							
Total Calories/Day							

1,000-Calorie Food Plan/Weekly Caloric Intake Diary

	Monday (Breakfast / Lunch / Dinner / Snack)	Tuesday	Wednesday	Thursday	Friday	Saturday	Sunday
1. Vegetable Exchanges A any amount B 25 calories	AA ○○	AA ○○	AA ○○	AA ○○	AA ○○	AA ○○	AA ○○
2. Fruit Exchanges 40 calories	○○○	○○○	○○○	○○○	○○○	○○○	○○○
3. Bread Exchanges 70 calories	○○○	○○○	○○○	○○○	○○○	○○○	○○○
4. Meat Exchanges 75 calories	○○○ ○	○○○ ○	○○○ ○	○○○ ○	○○○ ○	○○○ ○	○○○ ○
5. Milk Exchanges 80 calories	○ ○	○	○	○	○	○	○
6. Fats, Sweets and Beverages Exchanges 45 calories	○○○	○○○	○○○	○○○	○○○	○○○	○○○
7. Unlimited Exchanges 0 calories	AA	AA	AA	AA	AA	AA	AA
Food Exchange Calories							
Additional Calories							
Total Calories/Day							

1,200 -Calorie Food Plan/Weekly Caloric Intake Diary

	Monday	Tuesday	Wednesday	Thursday	Friday	Saturday	Sunday
	Breakfast / Lunch / Dinner / Snack	Breakfast / Lunch / Dinner / Snack	Breakfast / Lunch / Dinner / Snack	Breakfast / Lunch / Dinner / Snack	Breakfast / Lunch / Dinner / Snack	Breakfast / Lunch / Dinner / Snack	Breakfast / Lunch / Dinner / Snack
1. Vegetable Exchanges A any amount B 25 calories	AA OO	AA OO	AA OO	AA OO	AA OO	AA OO	AA OO
2. Fruit Exchanges 40 calories	OOO	OOO	OOO	OOO	OOO	OOO	OOO
3. Bread Exchanges 70 calories	OOO O	OOO O	OOO O	OOO O	OOO O	OOO O	OOO O
4. Meat Exchanges 75 calories	O OOO	O OOO	O OOO	OOO OOO	OOO OOO	OOO OOO	OOO OOO
5. Milk Exchanges 80 calories	O	O	O	O	O	O	O
6. Fats, Sweets and Beverages Exchanges 45 calories	OOOO	OOOO	OOOO	OOOO	OOOO	OOOO	OOOO
7. Unlimited Exchanges 0 calories	AA	AA	AA	AA	AA	AA	AA
Food Exchange Calories							
Additional Calories							
Total Calories/Day							

1,200-Calorie Food Plan/Weekly Caloric Intake Diary

Each day is divided into sub-columns: **Breakfast, Lunch, Dinner, Snack**.

	Monday (B/L/D/S)	Tuesday (B/L/D/S)	Wednesday (B/L/D/S)	Thursday (B/L/D/S)	Friday (B/L/D/S)	Saturday (B/L/D/S)	Sunday (B/L/D/S)
1. Vegetable Exchanges A any amount B 25 calories	A A / OO	A A / OO	A A / OO	A A / OO	A A / OO	A A / OO	A A / OO
2. Fruit Exchanges 40 calories	OOO	OOO	OOO	OOO	OOO	OOO	OOO
3. Bread Exchanges 70 calories	OO O / OOO	OO O / OOO	OOO / OOO	OO / OOO	OO / OOO	OO / OOO	OO / OOO
4. Meat Exchanges 75 calories	OO OOO	OO OOO	OO OOO	OO OOO	OO OOO	OO OOO	OO OOO
5. Milk Exchanges 80 calories	O	O	O	O	O	O	O
6. Fats, Sweets and Beverages Exchanges 45 calories	OOOO	OOOO	OOOO	OOOO	OOOO	OOOO	OOOO
7. Unlimited Exchanges 0 calories	A A	A A	A A	A A	A A	A A	A A
Food Exchange Calories							
Additional Calories							
Total Calories/Day							

1,500-Calorie Food Plan/Weekly Caloric Intake Diary

	Monday				Tuesday				Wednesday				Thursday				Friday				Saturday				Sunday			
	Breakfast	Lunch	Dinner	Snack	Breakfast	Lunch	Dinner	Snack	Breakfast	Lunch	Dinner	Snack	Breakfast	Lunch	Dinner	Snack	Breakfast	Lunch	Dinner	Snack	Breakfast	Lunch	Dinner	Snack	Breakfast	Lunch	Dinner	Snack
1. Vegetable Exchanges A any amount B 25 calories	A A	○	○ ○		A A	○	○ ○		A A	○	○ ○		A A	○	○ ○		A A	○	○ ○		A A	○	○ ○		A A	○	○ ○	
2. Fruit Exchanges 40 calories	○	○ ○	○		○	○ ○	○		○	○ ○	○		○	○ ○	○		○	○ ○	○		○	○ ○	○		○	○ ○	○	
3. Bread Exchanges 70 calories	○	○ ○	○ ○	○	○	○ ○	○ ○	○	○	○ ○	○ ○	○	○	○ ○	○ ○	○	○	○ ○	○ ○	○	○	○ ○	○ ○	○	○	○ ○	○ ○	○
4. Meat Exchanges 75 calories	○	○ ○	○ ○ ○		○	○ ○	○ ○ ○		○	○ ○	○ ○ ○		○	○ ○	○ ○ ○		○	○ ○	○ ○ ○		○	○ ○	○ ○ ○		○	○ ○	○ ○ ○	
5. Milk Exchanges 80 calories	○			○	○			○	○			○	○			○	○			○	○			○	○			○
6. Fats, Sweets and Beverages Exchanges 45 calories	○	○ ○	○ ○	○	○	○ ○	○ ○	○	○	○ ○	○ ○	○	○	○ ○	○ ○	○	○	○ ○	○ ○	○	○	○ ○	○ ○	○	○	○ ○	○ ○	○
7. Unlimited Exchanges 0 calories	A A				A A				A A				A A				A A				A A				A A			
Food Exchange Calories				—				—				—				—				—				—				—
Additional Calories				—				—				—				—				—				—				—
Total Calories/Day				—				—				—				—				—				—				—

1,500-Calorie Food Plan/Weekly Caloric Intake Diary

	Monday				Tuesday				Wednesday				Thursday				Friday				Saturday				Sunday			
	Breakfast	Lunch	Dinner	Snack	Breakfast	Lunch	Dinner	Snack	Breakfast	Lunch	Dinner	Snack	Breakfast	Lunch	Dinner	Snack	Breakfast	Lunch	Dinner	Snack	Breakfast	Lunch	Dinner	Snack	Breakfast	Lunch	Dinner	Snack
1. Vegetable Exchanges A any amount B 25 calories	A	A	○○		A	A	○○		A	A	○○		A	A	○○		A	A	○○		A	A	○○		A	A	○○	
2. Fruit Exchanges 40 calories	○	○○			○	○○○			○	○○○			○	○○○			○	○○○			○	○○○			○	○○○		
3. Bread Exchanges 70 calories	○○○○		○		○○○○		○		○○○○		○		○○○○		○		○○○○		○		○○○○		○		○○○○		○	
4. Meat Exchanges 75 calories	○○○	○○○			○○○	○○○			○○○	○○○			○○○	○○○			○	○○○	○○○		○○○	○○○			○○○	○○○		
5. Milk Exchanges 80 calories	○				○			○	○			○	○			○	○			○	○			○	○			○
6. Fats, Sweets and Beverages Exchanges 45 calories	○○○○	○○			○○○○		○		○○○○		○		○○○○		○		○○○○		○		○○○○		○		○○○○		○	
7. Unlimited Exchanges 0 calories	A	A			A	A			A	A			A	A			A	A			A	A			A	A		
Food Exchange Calories	—				—				—				—				—				—				—			
Additional Calories	—				—				—				—				—				—				—			
Total Calories/Day	—				—				—				—				—				—				—			

© Copyright 1977 by Prentice-Hall, Inc., Englewood Cliffs, N.J. 07632

1,800-Calorie Food Plan/Weekly Caloric Intake Diary

	Monday (B / L / D / S)	Tuesday (B / L / D / S)	Wednesday (B / L / D / S)	Thursday (B / L / D / S)	Friday (B / L / D / S)	Saturday (B / L / D / S)	Sunday (B / L / D / S)
1. Vegetable Exchanges A any amount B 25 calories	A A	A A	A A	A A	A A	A A	A A
2. Fruit Exchanges 40 calories	○ ○ ○	○ ○ ○	○ ○ ○	○ ○ ○	○ ○ ○	○ ○ ○	○ ○ ○
3. Bread Exchanges 70 calories	○ ○ ○ ○	○ ○ ○ ○	○ ○ ○	○ ○ ○	○ ○ ○	○ ○ ○	○ ○ ○
4. Meat Exchanges 75 calories	○ ○ ○ ○	○ ○ ○	○ ○ ○	○ ○ ○	○ ○ ○	○ ○ ○	○ ○ ○
5. Milk Exchanges 80 calories	○ ○	○ ○	○ ○	○ ○	○ ○	○ ○	○ ○
6. Fats, Sweets and Beverages Exchanges 45 calories	○ ○ ○	○ ○ ○	○ ○ ○ ○	○ ○ ○	○ ○ ○	○ ○ ○	○ ○ ○
7. Unlimited Exchanges 0 calories	A A	A A	A A	A A	A A	A A	A A
Food Exchange Calories	— —	— —	— —	— —	— —	— —	— —
Additional Calories	— —	— —	— —	— —	— —	— —	— —
Total Calories/Day	— —	— —	— —	— —	— —	— —	— —

© Copyright 1977 by Prentice-Hall, Inc., Englewood Cliffs, N.J. 07632

1,800-Calorie Food Plan/Weekly Caloric Intake Diary

	Monday				Tuesday				Wednesday				Thursday				Friday				Saturday				Sunday			
	B	L	D	S	B	L	D	S	B	L	D	S	B	L	D	S	B	L	D	S	B	L	D	S	B	L	D	S
1. Vegetable Exchanges A any amount B 25 calories	A	A			A	A			A	A			A	A			A	A			A	A			A	A		
2. Fruit Exchanges 40 calories	O	O	O		O	O	O		O	O	O		O	O	O		O	O	O		O	O	O		O	O	O	
3. Bread Exchanges 70 calories	OOO	OOO	OOO	OO	O	OOO	OOOO	OO	O	OO	OOO	OO	O	OO	OOO	OO	O	OO	OOO	OO	O	OO	OOO	OO	O	OO	OOO	OO
4. Meat Exchanges 75 calories	OO	OO	OOO		O	OOO	OOO		O	OOO	OOO		O	OOO	OOO		O	OOO	OOO		O	OOO	OOO		O	OOO	OOO	
5. Milk Exchanges 80 calories	O			O	O		O		O			O	O			O	O			O	O			O	O			O
6. Fats, Sweets and Beverages Exchanges 45 calories	OOOO	OOO			OOO	OOO			OOO	OOO			OO	OOO			OO	OOO			OO	OOO			OO	OOO		
7. Unlimited Exchanges 0 calories	A	A			A	A			A	A			A	A			A	A			A	A			A	A		
Food Exchange Calories																												
Additional Calories																												
Total Calories/Day																												

© Copyright 1977 by Prentice-Hall, Inc., Englewood Cliffs, N.J. 07632

Physical Activity Record

Physical Activity Record

Date	Physical Activity	Minutes Performed Activity	Calories Expended	Place: Home, Work Gym	People: Alone, Family Friends	Feelings

Physical Activity Record

Date	Physical Activity	Minutes Performed Activity	Calories Expended	Place: Home, Work Gym	People: Alone, Family Friends	Feelings

Physical Activity Record

Date	Physical Activity	Minutes Performed Activity	Calories Expended	Place: Home, Work Gym	People: Alone, Family Friends	Feelings

Appendix **G**

Weekly Physical Activity Diary

Weekly Physical Activity Diary

(A) 10-minute blocks	(B) Activity	(C) Calories per minute	(D) Blocks ×10 min.	(E) Total Calories Expended
	#1			
	#2			
	#3			
	#4			
	#5			

(1) Add right hand column to obtain total calories expended per week   = _____

(2) Divide by 3,500 calories to obtain pounds lost per week from physical activity   = _____

Weekly Physical Activity Diary

(A) 10-minute blocks	(B) Activity	(C) Calories per minute	(D) Blocks × 10 min.	(E) Total Calories Expended
	#1			
	#2			
	#3			
	#4			
	#5			

(1) Add right hand column to obtain total calories expended per week   = _____

(2) Divide by 3,500 calories to obtain pounds lost per week from physical activity   = _____

Caloric Intake, Caloric Expenditure, And Weight Loss Graph

Caloric Intake, Caloric Expenditure, and Weight Loss Graph

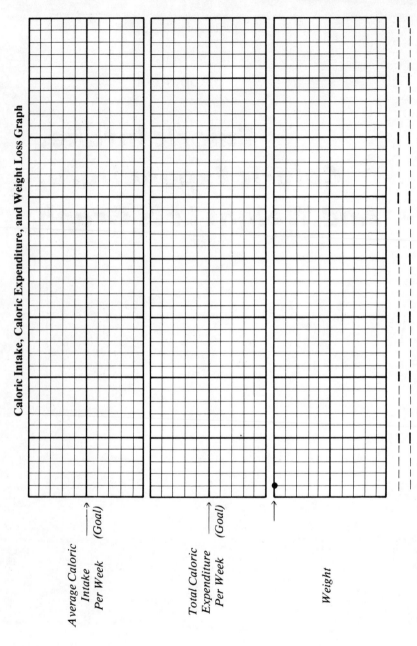

Average Caloric
Intake
Per Week
———→
(Goal)

Total Caloric
Expenditure
Per Week
———→
(Goal)

Weight

Caloric Intake, Caloric Expenditure, and Weight Loss Graph

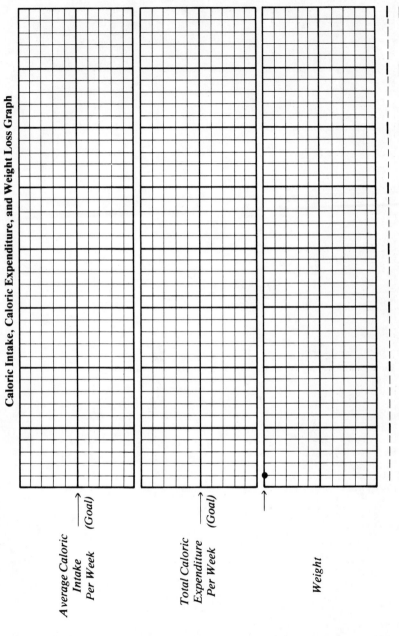

Average Caloric Intake Per Week ——→ *(Goal)*

Total Caloric Expenditure Per Week ——→ *(Goal)*

Weight

Weekly Weight Graphs

Weekly Weight Graph

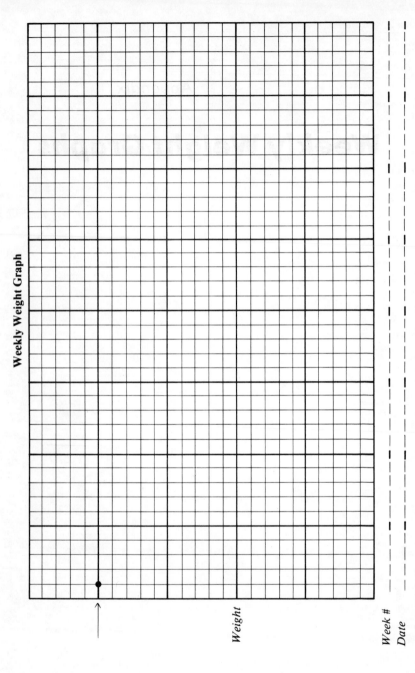

Weight

Week #

Date

Weekly Weight Graph

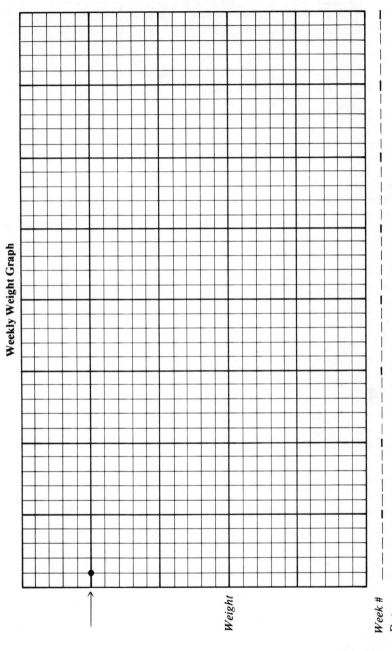

Weight

Appendix J

Behavioral Contract for Weight Management

This agreement, made and entered into this_____day of_____, 19____, by and between_____and_____.

Witnesseth:

A. *My Weight Management Goals:*

I,_____, have reviewed various possible weight management goals and have agreed to work hard at achieving the following, realistic goals. (Check off and fill in the details of only the goals that will be helpful to *you*.)

1. I will seek to lose between____and____pounds per week and continue to lose weight until I reach my weight goal of____pounds.

2. I will observe regularly my
   a. caloric intake   Yes____   No____
   b. caloric expenditure   Yes____   No____
   c. weekly weight   Yes____   No____

3. I will keep my caloric intake, on the average, at_____calories or less.

4. I will increase my weekly physical activities
   a. To use up_____or more calories per week
   b. To do one or more of the following activities
      (1)_____   (3)_____
      (2)_____   (4)_____

5. I agree to work on the following eating habits
   a._____
   b._____
   c._____

6. I also agree to work on the following habit changes: (fill in any additional goals you want to achieve)
   a._____
   b._____
   c._____

B.   *My Rewards and Consequences*

(Check off and fill in the details of only the consequences that will be helpful to *you.*)

1. I,_____, agree to make a total deposit of $_____. I further agree to pay myself $_____ of the total deposit each week I achieve my habit improvement and weight loss goals. If I do not make my weight improvement goals, I agree *not* to pay myself that week. Any money not earned back by the end of the program will be given to _____.

2. I will reward myself weekly with one or more of the following activities. (List rewarding activities.)
   a._____
   b._____
   c._____
   d._____
   e._____

3. My weight management partner, _____, agrees to do the following when I make my weekly goals.
   a. Praise me for my efforts
   b. Do the following for me _____
   _____

4. When I do *not* make my weekly goals I agree to do the following:
   _____
   _____

5. Additional Consequences: _____
   _____

We have both read the above contract and agree to the goals and consequences checked. We both agree to follow the contract until the goals or review date are reached, whichever comes first. We may at that time renegotiate the contract.

First Partner:_____   Second Partner:_____

Current Date:_____

Review Date:_____

BEHAVIORAL CONTRACT FOR WEIGHT MANAGEMENT

This agreement, made and entered into this_____day of_____, 19____, by and between_____and_____.

Witnesseth:

A. *My Weight Management Goals:*

I,_____, have reviewed various possible weight management goals and have agreed to work hard at achieving the following, realistic goals. (Check off and fill in the details of only the goals that will be helpful to *you*.)

1. I will seek to lose between____and____pounds per week and continue to lose weight until I reach my weight goal of____pounds.

2. I will observe regularly my
   a. caloric intake   Yes____   No____
   b. caloric expenditure   Yes____   No____
   c. weekly weight   Yes____   No____

3. I will keep my caloric intake, on the average, at_____calories or less.

4. I will increase my weekly physical activities
   a. To use up____or more calories per week
   b. To do one or more of the following activities
      (1) _____   (3) _____
      (2) _____   (4) _____

5. I agree to work on the following eating habits
   a. _____
   b. _____
   c. _____

6. I also agree to work on the following habit changes: (fill in any additional goals you want to achieve)
   a. _____
   b. _____
   c. _____

B. *My Rewards and Consequences*

(Check off and fill in the details of only the consequences that will be helpful to *you*.)
1. I,_____, agree to make a total deposit of $_____. I further agree to pay myself $_____ of the total deposit each week I achieve

my habit improvement and weight loss goals. If I do not make my weight improvement goals, I agree *not* to pay myself that week. Any money not earned back by the end of the program will be given to

_____.

2. I will reward myself weekly with one or more of the following activities. (List rewarding activities.)
   a. _____
   b. _____
   c. _____
   d. _____
   e. _____

3. My weight management partner,_____, agrees to do the following when I make my weekly goals.
   a. Praise me for my efforts
   b. Do the following for me _____
   _____

4. When I do *not* make my weekly goals I agree to do the following:
   _____
   _____

5. Additional Consequences: _____
   _____

We have both read the above contract and agree to the goals and consequences checked. We both agree to follow the contract until the goals or review date are reached, whichever comes first. We may at that time renegotiate the contract.

First Partner: _____   Second Partner:_____
Current Date:_____

Review Date: _____

Appendix

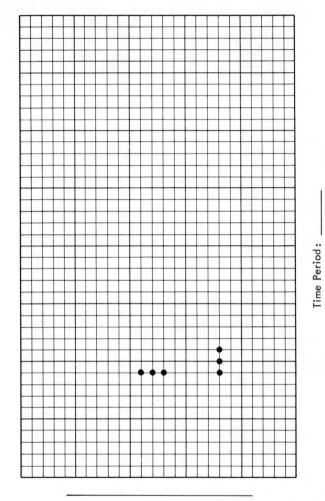

Eating or Exercising Behavior:

Time Period: _____

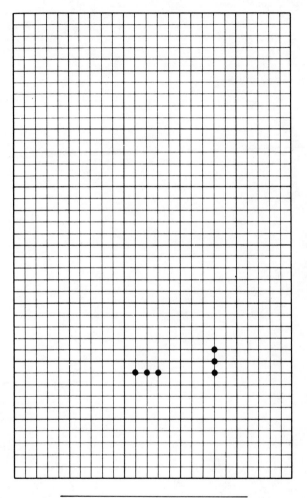

Eating or Exercising Behavior:

Time Period: _____

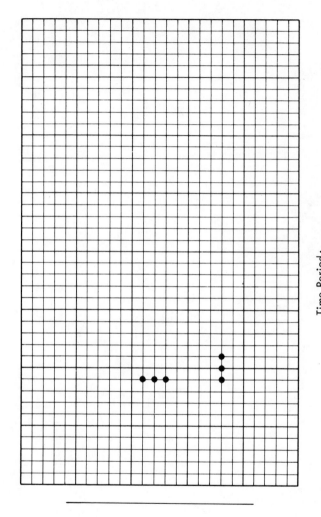

Time Period : _____

Eating or Exercising Behavior: _____

References

The reference lists include articles and books that supplement the material in the book. These references are not exclusive of the area, but hopefully they will provide a start for the reader who is interested in a more thorough understanding of the field.

A. BEHAVIOR MODIFICATION AND THERAPY

Abramson, E. D. A review of behavioral approaches to weight control. *Behaviour Research and Therapy,* 1973, *11,* 547–556.

Alberti, R. E. and M. L. Emmons. *Yoar perfect right: A guide to assertive behavior.* San Luis Obispo, Ca: Impract Pub., 1974.

Bandura, A. *Principles of behavior modification.* New York: Holt, Rinehart & Winston, 1969.

Becker, W. *Parents are teachers.* Champaign, Ill.: Research Press, 1973.

Bellack, A. S. Behavior therapy for weight reduction: an evaluative review. *Addictive Behaviors,* in press.

Bowers, S. and G. Bowers. *Asserting yourself.* New York: Addison Wesley, 1976.

Cautela, J. R. The treatment of over-eating by covert conditioning. *Psychotherapy: Theory, Research and Practice,* 1972, *9,* 211–216.

Chapman, S. Situational management, self-standard setting, and self-reward in a weight loss group. Unpublished doctoral dissertation. Emory University, Atlanta, 1976.

Christensen, E. R., D. B. Jeffrey, and J. P. Pappas. A therapist manual for a behavior modification weight reduction program. In E. E. Abramson, ed., *Behavioral programs for the treatment of obesity.* New York: Springer, 1977.

DeRisi, W. and G. Butz, *Writing behavioral contracts.* Champaign, Ill.: Research Press, 1974.

Ferster, C. B., J. E. Nurnberger and E. B. Levitt. The control of eating. *Journal of Mathetics,* 1962, *1,* 87–109.

Foreyt, J. P., ed. *Behavior modification approaches to obesity.* New York: Pergamon, 1977.

Goldfried, M. R. and M. Merbaum, eds. *Behavioral change through self-control.* New York: Holt, Rinehart & Winston, 1973.

Hagen, R. L. Group therapy versus bibliotherapy in weight reduction. *Behavior Therapy,* 1974, *5,* 222–234.

Hall, S. M. Self-control and therapist control in the behavioral treatment of overweight women. *Behaviour Research and Therapy,* 1972, *10,* 59–68.

————, and R. G. Hall. Outcome and methodological considerations in behavioral treatment of obesity. *Behavior Therapy,* 1974, *5,* 352–364.

Harmatz, M. G. and P. Lapuc. Behavior modification of overeating in a psychiatric population. *Journal of Consulting and Clinical Psychology,* 1968, *32,* 583–587.

Harris, M. B. Self-directed program for weight control: A pilot study. *Journal of Abnormal Psychology,* 1969, 74, 263–270.

_____ and C. G. Bruner. A comparison of a self-control and a contract procedure for weight control. *Behaviour Research and Therapy,* 1971, *9,* 347–354.

Homme, C. *How to use contingency contracting in the classroom.* Champaign, Ill.: Research Press, 1969.

Jeffrey, D. B. Self-control: Methodological issues and research trends. In M. J. Mahoney and C. E. Thoresen, eds., *Self-control: Power to the person.* Belmont, Ca.: Brooks/Cole, 1974. pp. 166–199.

_____. A comparison of the effects of external control and self-control on the modification and maintenance of weight. *Journal of Abnormal Psychology,* 1974, *83,* 404–410.

_____. Some methodological issues in research on obesity. *Psychological Reports,* 1974, *35,* 623–626.

_____. External vs. self-control in the management and maintenance of weight loss. In R. C. Katz and S. Zlutnick, eds., *Behavior therapy and health care: Principles and applications.* New York: Pergamon, 1975.

_____. Treatment evaluation issues in research on addictive behaviors. *Addictive Behaviors,* 1975, *1,* 23–36.

_____. Additional methodological considerations in the behavioral treatment of obesity: A reply to the Hall and Hall review of obesity. *Behavior Therapy,* 1975, *6,* 96–97.

_____. Behavioral management of obesity. In W. E. Craighead, A. E. Kazdin, and M. J. Mahoney, eds., *Behavior modification: Principles, Issues and applications.* New York: Houghton Mifflin, 1976.

_____. A proposal for a macro environmental analysis in the prevention and treatment of obesity. In B. J. Williams, S. Martin, and J. P. Foreyt, eds., *Obesity: behavioral approaches to dietary management.* New York: Brunner/Mazel, 1976.

_____. Treatment outcome issues in obesity research. In B. J. Williams, S. Martin, and J. P. Foreyt, eds., *Obesity: Behavioral approaches to dietary management.* New York: Brunner/Mazel, 1976.

_____. Self-control approaches in the management of obesity. In J. P. Foreyt, ed., *Behavior modification approaches to obesity.* New York: Pergamon, 1977.

_____, and E. R. Christensen. Behavior therapy versus "will power" in the management of obesity. *Journal of Psychology,* 1975, *90,* 303–311.

_____, E. R. Christensen, and R. C. Katz. Behavior therapy weight reduction programs: Some preliminary findings on the need for follow-ups. *Psychotherapy: Therapy, Research and Practice,* 1975, *90,* 303–311.

_____, E. R. Christensen, and J. P. Pappas. Developing a behavioral program and therapist manual for the treatment of obesity. *Journal of the American College Health Association,* 1973, *21,* 455–459.

Katz, R. C. and S. Zlutnick, eds. *Behavior therapy and health care: Principles and applications.* New York: Pergamon, 1975.

Knox, G. Ten misconceptions about overweight and dieting. *Better Homes and Gardens,* 1972, June, 12–13.

Levitz, L. and A. Stunkard. A therapeutic condition for obesity: Behavior modification and patient self-help. *American Journal of Psychiatry,* 1974, *131,* 423–427.

Lutzker, S. and J. Lutzker. A two-dimensional marital contract: Weight loss and household responsibility performance. Paper presented at meeting of the Western Psychological Association, 1974.

Mahoney, M. J. Self-reward and self-monitoring techniques for weight control. *Behavior Therapy,* 1974, *5,* 48–57.

_____, and D. B. Jeffrey. A manual of self-control procedures for the overweight. *Catalog of Selected Documents in Psychology,* 1974, *4,* 129.

_____, N. G. Moura, and T. C. Wade. Relative efficacy of self-reward, self-punishment and self-monitoring techniques for weight loss. *Journal of Consulting and Clinical Psychology,* 1973, *40,* 404–407.

McReynolds, W. T., R. N. Lutz, B. K. Paulsen, and M. B. Kohrs. Weight loss resulting from two behavior modification procedures with nutritionists as therapists. *Behavior Therapy,* 1976, *7,* 283–291.

Miller, P. M. The use of behavioral contracting in the treatment of alcoholism: a case study. *Behavior Therapy,* 1972, *3,* 593–596.

Patterson, G. *Families.* Champaign, Ill.: Research Press, 1974.

Penick, S. B., R. Filion, S. Fox, and A. J. Stunkard. Behavior modification in the treatment of obesity. *Psychosomatic Medicine,* 1971, *33,* 49–55.

Schacter, S. *Emotions, obesity and crime.* New York: Academic Press, 1971.

Skinner, B. *About behaviorism.* New York: Alfred Knopf, 1974.

Stuart, R. B. Behavioral control of over-eating. *Behavior Research and Therapy,* 1967, *5,* 357–365.

————. A three-dimensional program for the treatment of obesity. *Behaviour Research and Therapy,* 1971, *9,* 177–186.

————, and B. Davis. *Slim chance in a fat world: Behavioral control of obesity.* Champaign, Ill.: Research Press, 1972.

Stunkard, A. J. and M. J. Mahoney. Behavioral treatment of the eating disorders. In H. Leitenberg, ed., *Handbook of behavior modification.* New York: Appleton-Century-Crofts, 1976.

Thoresen, C. E. and M. J. Mahoney. *Behavioral self-control.* New York: Holt, Rinehart & Winston, 1974.

Williams, B. J., S. Martin, and J. P. Foreyt, eds., *Obesity: behavioral approaches to dietary management.* New York: Brunner/Mazel, 1976.

Wollersheim, P. Effectiveness of group therapy based upon learning principles in the treatment of overweight women. *Journal of Abnormal Psychology,* 1970, *76,* 462–474.

B. GENERAL

Berland, T. *Rating the diets*. Skokie, Ill.: Comsumer Guide, 1974.

Dallas Independent School District, Administration Code 2480.5. Dallas, Texas, 1975.

Eden, A. *Growing up thin*. New York: David McKay, 1975.

Hirsch, J., J. L. Knittle, and L. B. Solans. Cell liped content and cell number in obese and non-obese human adipose tissue. *Journal of Clinical Investigation,* 1966, *45,* 1023.

Konishi, F. Food energy equivalents of activities. *Journal American Dietetic Association,* 1965, *46,* 186.

Mayer, J. *Overweight: causes, cost, and control*. Englewood Cliffs, N.J.: Prentice-Hall, 1968.

_____. *A diet for living*. New York: David McKay, 1975.

Ruben, D. *The save your life diet*. New York: Random House, 1975.

Stunkard, A. Obesity. In A. Freedman, H. Kaplan, and B. Sadock, eds. *Comprehensive textbook of psychiatry*. Baltimore: William and Wilkens, 1976, pp. 1648–1654.

_____. *The pain of obesity*. Palo Alto, Calif.: Bull Publishers, 1976.

United States Department of Agriculture. *Agricultural statistics*. United States Government Printing Office, 1973.

United States Public Health Service. *Obesity and health*. Washington, D. C., U. S. Government Printing Office, undated.

Wyden, P. *The overweight society*. New York: William Morrow, 1965.

C.   NUTRITION AND LOW-CALORIE COOK BOOKS

American Dietetic Association. *Exchange Lists for Meal Planning*. Chicago: American Dietetic Association, 1976.

American Heart Association. *The American Heart Association Cookbook.* New York: David McKay, 1973.

Better Homes and Gardens. *Calories counter's cookbook.* New York: Better Homes and Gardens Books, 1970.

Cutler, C. *Haute cuisine for your heart's delight: a low cholesterol cookbook for gourmets.* New York: Clarkson N. Potter, 1973.

Frances, E. *Ladies Home Journal Family diet book.* New York: Macmillan, 1973.

Fredericks, C. *The new and revised Carlton Fredericks cookbook for good nutrition.* New York: Grosset and Dunlap, 1974.

Kraus, B. *Calories and carbohydrates.* New York: New American Library, 1973.

Lappe, F. *Diet for a small planet.* New York: Ballantine, 1975.

United States Department of Agriculture. *Calories and weight.* Washington, D.C.: U. S. Government Printing Office, Home and Garden Bulletin No. 153, USDA, 1968.

D. PHYSICAL ACTIVITY AND EXERCISE

Back, L. *Awake! Aware! Alive! Exercise for a vital body.* New York: Random House, 1973.

Cooper, K. *Aerobics.* New York: Bantam, 1972.

Craig, M. *Miss Craig's 21-day shape-up program for men and women.* New York: Random House, 1968.

Durnin, J. U. G. A. and R. Passmore. *Energy work and leisure.* London: Heiremann Educational Books Ltd., 1967.

Hittleman, R. *Richard Hittleman's yoga 28 day exercise plan.* New York: Bantam, 1973.

Johnson, P. B., W. F. Updyke, M. Schaefer, and D. C. Stolberg. *Sports, exercise, and you.* New York: Holt, Rinehart & Winston, 1975.

Morehouse L. and L. Gross. *Total fitness in thirty minutes a week.* New York: Simon and Schuster, 1975.

E. SELF-MANAGEMENT SERIES

Heiman, J., L. LoPiccolo, and J. LoPiccolo. *Becoming orgasmic: a sexual growth program for women.* Englewood Cliffs, N.J.: Prentice-Hall, 1976.

Miller, W. R. and R. Munoz. *How to control your drinking.* Englewood Cliffs, N.J.: Prentice-Hall, 1976.

Rosen, G. *Don't be afraid: A program for overcoming fears and phobias.* Englewood Cliffs, N.J.: Prentice-Hall, 1977.

Thoresen, C. E. and T. J. Coates. *How to sleep better: A drug-free program for overcoming insomnia.* Englewood Cliffs, N.J.: Prentice-Hall, 1977.

Index

A

Alcohol, 177-78
Anorexia nervosa, 261

B

Baseline information, 242-46
Behavioral contracting:
   definition of, 209
   examples, 217 ff
   rules for, 214
Behavioral self-control, 38 ff
Buying food, 155

W

THE SELF-MANAGEMENT PSYCHOLOGY SERIES
Carl E. Thoresen, Ph.D., *General Editor*
Stanford University

This series of self-help books presents techniques that really work based on scientifically sound research.

Designed with the layman in mind, each book presents a step-by-step method you can readily apply to solve real problems you confront in everyday life. Each is written by a respected behavioral scientist who has achieved success in applying these same techniques.

D. BALFOUR JEFFREY is an assistant professor of clinical psychology at the University of Montana. ROGER C. KATZ is an assistant professor at the University of the Pacific.

BOOKS IN THE SERIES

How to Control Your Drinking,
by William R. Miller and Ricardo F. Muñoz

Becoming Orgasmic: A Sexual Growth Program for Women,
by Julia Heiman, Leslie LoPiccolo, and Joseph LoPiccolo

How to Sleep Better: A Drug-Free Program for Overcoming Insomnia, by Thomas Coates and Carl E. Thoresen

How to Become an Ex-Smoker, by Carl E. Thoresen

Take It Off and Keep It Off: A Behavioral Program for Weight Loss and Exercise, by D. Balfour Jeffrey and Roger C. Katz

Don't Be Afraid: A Program for Overcoming Fears and Phobias,
by Gerald Rosen